高等医学院校实验教材

供临床、预防、护理、口腔、麻醉等医学类专业使用

机能实验学教程与强化训练

Course of Functional Experiment Science and Intensive Training

主　编　杨秀红　张连元

副主编　王艳蕾　赵利军　白　静　韩淑英
　　　　门秀丽　段国贤

编　者　（按姓名汉语拼音排序）

安春娜　白　静　储金秀　段国贤
耿　菲　勾向博　韩　婷　韩淑英
李　颖　李树民　刘　燕　门秀丽
秦丽娟　孙　娜　王建辉　王树华
王小君　王艳蕾　王银环　吴　静
薛　涛　杨秀红　张　娜　张　田
张　伟　张博男　张连元　张一兵
赵利军　朱丽艳　Daniel H. Nissen

北京大学医学出版社

图书在版编目（CIP）数据

机能实验学教程与强化训练/杨秀红，张连元主编.
—北京：北京大学医学出版社，2014.2（2019.7重印）
ISBN 978-7-5659-0730-2

Ⅰ.①机⋯　Ⅱ.①杨⋯　②张⋯　Ⅲ.①实验医学—医学
院校—教材　Ⅳ.①R-33

中国版本图书馆 CIP 数据核字（2013）第 308825 号

机能实验学教程与强化训练

主　　编：杨秀红　张连元
出版发行：北京大学医学出版社
地　　址：（100191）北京市海淀区学院路 38 号　北京大学医学部院内
电　　话：发行部 010 - 82802230；图书邮购 010 - 82802495
网　　址：http：//www. pumpress. com. cn
E - mail：booksale@bjmu. edu. cn
印　　刷：北京溢漾印刷有限公司
经　　销：新华书店
责任编辑：罗德刚　金美娜　　**责任校对**：金彤文　　　**责任印制**：罗德刚
开　　本：787mm×1092mm　1/16　　**印张**：10.5　　**字数**：264 千字
版　　次：2014 年 2 月第 1 版　2019 年 7 月第 6 次印刷
书　　号：ISBN 978-7-5659-0730-2
定　　价：22.00 元

版权所有，违者必究
（凡属质量问题请与本社发行部联系退换）

前　言

机能实验学将生理学、病理生理学和药理学三门学科的实验内容有机地融合在一起，用实验的方法来观察和研究正常、疾病状态以及药物作用下机体的功能活动规律，其目标是培养学生较强的综合分析能力、开拓创新意识和科学思维方式。

目前，各高校机能实验的条件、设备、技术力量不尽相同，开设实验的学时、内容和考核方式也没有统一的标准。由于本学科涉及的实验内容比较广泛，使用动物种类多，有些实验操作难度较大，即使学生课前预习实验内容，老师课堂耐心指导，也常常会出现实验失败现象。为学生提供一本内容丰富、结构严谨、实用性强的机能实验教材，以提高机能实验教学水平，达到机能实验学的培养目标，是从事机能实验教学研究的高校教师应尽的责任和义务。为此，我们根据自身实验条件和学生实际需要，编写了这本《机能实验学教程与强化训练》实验教材。

按照课程的实施过程，本教材共分七章。第一章是绪论，主要介绍了机能实验学的基本概念、教学内容和基本要求。第二章描述了计算机生物机能实验系统等机能实验常用仪器和设备。第三章内容涉及实验动物的基本知识和操作技能。上述三章内容使学生掌握机能实验的基本理论知识和基本技术，在此基础之上，我们将三门学科经典的动物实验教学内容进行衔接，有意识地进行融合和相互渗透，归为第四章，即基础和综合性实验。第五章紧密结合临床实践，编写了便于操作的人体机能实验，为提高学生的临床技能打下基础。第六章为设计性实验教学内容，在介绍实验选题、设计、实施和论文撰写内容之后，根据本校机能学科的研究方向，列举部分设计性实验参考项目，启迪学生的思维，供对相关领域研究感兴趣的学生选择，为他们参加大学生创新性实验计划提供参考。此外，根据机能学科留学生实验教学的需要，教材中"常用实验动物与动物实验基本知识""基础及综合性实验""人体机能实验"这三章的大部分内容采取了中英文对照的形式，这是本教材编写的一大特色。

为了尽快提高学生的动手操作能力、分析和解决问题能力及创新思维能力，提高实验的成功率，编者深入课堂，从学生的角度针对实验提出相关问题，包括实验原理和相关理论、实验操作和技术等内容，编写了 7 套机能实验习题及解答，方便学生课后训练。

本教材的编写得到了我校基础医学院领导的大力支持，在此表示衷心感谢。由于编者水平有限，内容涉及学科较多，虽经过多次讨论和审阅，缺点和错误在所难免，恳请同仁和读者批评指正，以便再版时修订和完善。我们真诚地希望，这本书能为学生和教师提供更加切实有效的帮助。

杨秀红　张连元

2013 年 11 月

目　录

第一章 绪 论

第一节 机能实验学概述

机能实验学（Functional experiment science）是研究生物体功能活动规律的实验性学科。它包括生理学研究的正常机体功能活动规律，病理生理学研究的疾病状态下机体的功能活动规律和药理学研究的药物作用对机体正常或异常功能活动规律的影响等。它将正常生命活动、疾病、药物干预有机结合，强调学科之间的交叉融合，便于学生系统了解生命活动的正常生理、疾病发生发展和药物防治的基本规律及特征，形成对机体功能代谢变化的完整认识，同时注重培养和提高学生的创新、动手、分析和解决问题的能力。

一、机能实验学及其任务

（一）机能实验学概念

机能实验学是一门综合性的实验课程，融汇了生理学、病理生理学与药理学三门课程的实验内容，研究内容包括生物体正常生理功能和疾病发生发展过程中的规律与发病机制，分析和探讨药物在体内的代谢和作用。

（二）培养目标

通过本课程的学习，使学生直观地认识人体功能基本理论；初步掌握科学研究中常用的方法、手段和实验设计思路；培养学生科学的思维能力和创新意识，养成理论联系实际和勇于探索的科学精神。具体目标如下。

1. 综合运用生理学、病理生理学与药理学相关知识，加深对人体功能基本理论的理解。

2. 熟悉和掌握机能实验常用仪器、设备的使用方法和动物实验的基本知识。

3. 了解和掌握人体机能学研究的常用方法和技术，掌握动物实验的基本操作技能，了解科学研究的基本思路与方法。

4. 学会实验资料的收集、整理和数据处理及对实验结果的分析、讨论，提高学生综合分析问题和解决问题的能力，从而培养严谨的科学作风和严密的逻辑思维能力。

（三）教学内容

这门课程除了将原生理学、病理生理学、药理学的经典教学实验归纳为基础性实验外，还比较系统地增加了实验基本知识、实验基本方法和操作技能等方面的内容，同时将上述三门学科的实验进行有机整合，形成了综合性实验项目和设计性实验内容。教学内容主要包括以下几个方面：

1. 常用实验仪器的工作原理和使用方法，常用动物实验的技术操作。

2. 基础实验，包括整体动物或动物的离体组织、器官的正常和异常生理活动的观察和记录，及某些药物对这些动物或离体组织生理功能的影响。

3. 综合性实验，观察单因素或多因素对动物生理功能活动的影响，分析其功能变化发生的可能机制，掌握有效的处理方法并了解其可能的作用机制。

4. 人体机能实验，观察人体细胞、器官、系统乃至整体水平所表现的各种生命现象、活动规律，了解人体与环境之间的相互作用、健康以及维持健康的基本知识。

5. 设计性实验，在学生掌握了机能实验学相关理论和基本实验方法的基础上，在老师的指导下，学生自行完成实验设计、实验准备、实验操作以及实验数据的收集、整理及撰写实验报告。

二、机能实验学分类

机能实验的观察对象包括人体和实验动物。

（一）人体实验

在人（健康人或患者）身上进行的、以取得实验者所需资料的实验称为人体实验。这类实验对人体无损伤或损伤极小，操作简单易行，方法容易掌握，能多次重复，便于动态观察（如视野和盲点的测定）。通过在正常人体测定一些客观指标，来计算这些指标在正常人群的变化范围和正常平均值等项目，用于衡量人体的健康状况；对病态机体进行测量，以协助临床诊断，了解疾病的进展和治疗效果。

（二）动物实验

机能实验学以动物实验为主，根据实验目的的不同，可以采取不同的实验方法，主要包括以下两个方面。

1. 急性实验　在短时间内完成整体动物或离体器官、组织的功能活动观察和记录即为急性实验，是机能实验常用的方法。分为离体实验和在体实验。主要优点是实验条件比较简单，不需严格的无菌操作，不在实验范围内的许多其他条件一般均可被人工控制，并有可能对观察对象的某种功能进行直接的观察和细致的分析。主要缺点是由于时间短和对整体功能不可避免的破坏，难以获取全面的资料和进行动态的观察。

2. 慢性实验　慢性实验以完整、健康的动物为对象，且尽可能保持外界环境接近于自然，以便能在较长时间内反复多次观察和记录机体某些功能的改变。主要优点是可以长时间地动态观察，便于全面、系统地对实验动物的功能、代谢活动进行综合研究分析。主要缺点是实验观察时间长，实验条件难于控制。

（刘　燕）

第二节　实验报告的书写要求

实验报告的书写是一项重要的基本技能训练，有助于提高综合分析能力及逻辑思考能力。书写报告应注意结构完整、文字简练、条理清楚，并注意科学性和逻辑性。完整的实验报告应包括以下项目：

1. 一般信息　姓名，年级，班次，组别，实验日期（年、月、日）和室温等。

2. 实验名称　高度概括实验内容，用语要准确、明白，符合科学规范。

3. 实验目的　主要说明通过实验验证有关理论，以及所要达到的预期结果。

4. 实验原理　是指实验设计的依据和思路。根据不同的实验可以进行文字叙述，也可用计算公式、化学反应方程式表达。

5. 实验对象　应注明实验对象的种属、性别、体重、数量。

6. 实验用品　是指实验所使用的主要的仪器、器械和试剂。

7. 实验步骤　简要写出实验效应指标的观察方法、手术操作过程、标本的制备、记录手段及注意事项等。

8. 实验结果　是指实验材料经实验过程加工处理后得到的结果。它是实验结论的依据，整个实验报告的核心。根据实验目的将原始记录系统化、条理化。其表达方式一般有 3 种：

（1）叙述式：用文字将观察到的与实验目的有关的现象客观地加以描述。描述时需要有时间顺序。

（2）表格式：能较为清楚地反映观察内容，使实验结果突出、清楚，便于相互比较。每一表格应说明一定的中心问题，应标有栏头和计量单位。

（3）简图式：实验中观察到的各种指标如血压、呼吸、心室内压等，可用曲线图表示，也可取其不同的时相点，用直线图表示。此法使其形象生动，一目了然。

若 3 种表达方式并用，可得到最佳的效果，报告的质量也将明显提高。

9. 分析与讨论　讨论主要是针对实验中所观察到的现象与结果，联系理论知识对其进行分析研究和解释，得出必要的结论。这部分是实验结果的逻辑延伸，是实验报告的主体。讨论内容包括：

（1）以实验结果为论据，论证实验目的。

（2）根据已知的理论知识对结果进行解释和分析。

（3）如实验出现了非预期的结果，应该考虑和分析其原因。

10. 实验结论　实验结论是实验报告最终的总体上的总结，即是从"结果"和"讨论"中归纳出来的概括性判断。不要罗列具体的经过或重复讨论的内容。结论的文字要精练。

（刘　燕）

第三节　实验课的基本要求与注意事项

一、基本要求

（一）实验前

1. 预习实验教材，明确本次实验的目的、要求、步骤，充分理解本次实验的意义。

2. 设计好实验原始记录的表格，对本实验结果做出初步科学预测并加以分析。

3. 熟悉所用仪器的性能及手术的基本操作方法。

4. 检查实验器材和药品是否齐全、完好。

5. 注意和估计实验中可能发生的误差并制定防止误差的方法。

（二）实验中

1. 实验室应保持安静和清洁，不得进行与实验无关的活动。

2. 小组成员既要有明确分工，又要注意团结合作，这样既可提高实验的成功率，又能使每个同学都能得到应有的技能训练。

3. 按照实验步骤，以严肃认真的态度循序操作，不得随意变动，要注意保护实验动物和标本，爱护并节省实验器材和药品。

4. 仔细、耐心地观察实验过程中出现的现象，随时记录并联系讲授内容进行思考。如实验取得了什么结果？为什么出现这种结果？这种结果的意义是什么？根据相关理论解释出现这些结果的原因，并和小组成员之间进行深入的讨论。

（三）实验后

1. 清点并清洗实验器材，如有器械损坏或遗失，要立即报告负责教师。

2. 整理实验结果，认真撰写实验报告。实验结果必须真实、准确、可靠。

3. 实验报告应按时上交，评阅后的报告应妥善保存，期末时全部上交并存档。

4. 把实验废弃物品、动物尸体及存活动物分类集中放到指定地点，严禁乱放乱弃。

5. 安排值日生搞好实验室清洁卫生，离开实验室前应关好电源、水龙头和门窗。

二、注意事项

（一）文明守时

遵守纪律，准时到达实验室（值日生应提早 20 min），在室内应穿白大衣。

（二）安静有序

进入实验室应服从教师指导，在指定的位置做实验，不得在室内喧哗、打闹；不得将与实验无关的物品带入实验室，未经允许不得将实验室物品带出实验室。

（三）严守规矩

严格按仪器操作规程进行操作，如仪器失灵、损坏、器材不足等，应及时报告；如有不应有的损坏及过量消耗，按照具体情况由个人或小组赔偿。

（四）善待动物

进行动物实验时，要正确抓取动物，禁止粗暴捕捉，以免被动物咬伤或造成动物伤亡和应激反应。必须对动物有爱心，不要增加动物不必要的痛苦。若被动物咬伤，应立即将血液挤出，清水冲洗，以碘酊消毒。

（李　颖）

第二章　常用仪器和器械的使用

第一节　BL-420生物机能实验系统

一、BL-420生物机能实验系统软、硬件组成

BL-420生物机能实验系统是配置在计算机上的4通道生物信号采集、放大、显示、记录与处理系统。它由以下3个主要部分构成：计算机、BL-420系统硬件和BL-420生物信号显示与处理软件，如图2-1所示。

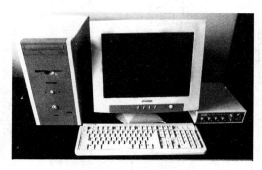

图2-1　BL-420生物机能实验系统组成
Fig. 2-1　Composition of BL-420 data acquisition and analysis system

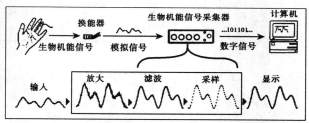

图2-2　BL-420生物机能实验系统原理图
Fig. 2-2　Principle of BL-420 data acquisition and analysis system

二、BL-420生物机能实验系统基本原理

首先将原始的生物机能信号，包括生物电信号和通过传感器引入的生物非电信号进行放大、滤波等处理；然后对处理的信号通过模数转换进行数字化，并将数字化后的生物机能信号传输到计算机内部，计算机则通过专用的生物机能实验系统软件接收从生物信号放大、采集卡传入的数字信号；然后对这些收到的信号进行实时处理，一方面进行生物机能波形的显示，另一方面进行生物机能信号的存贮，如图2-2所示。

三、BL-420系统软件界面及各部分功能介绍

（一）BL-420生物信号显示与处理软件主界面
如图2-3所示，从上到下依次主要由标题条、菜单条、工具条、时间显示窗口、波形

显示窗口和状态条等组成；从左到右依次为标尺调节区、左侧和右侧波形显示窗口、分时复用区等。此外，左上有刺激器调节区，左下有 Marker 标记区。

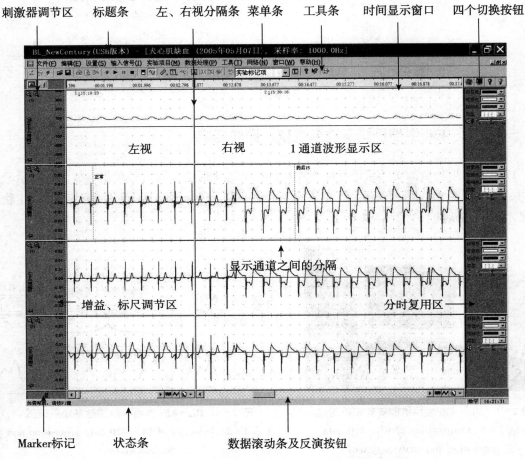

图 2 - 3　BL - 420 生物信号显示与处理软件主界面

Fig. 2 - 3　Graphical user interface of BL - 420 system

(二) BL - 420 软件主界面上常用菜单和按钮功能

1. "文件"菜单　"文件"菜单包含有"打开"、"另存为"、"退出"等 13 个命令。

2. "输入信号"菜单　"输入信号"菜单中包括有"1 通道"、"2 通道"、"3 通道"、"4 通道"共计 4 个选项，每个选项有一个输入信号选择子菜单，包括"动作电位"、"压力"等信号选项，如图 2 - 4 所示。

3. "实验项目"菜单　"实验项目"下拉式菜单中主要包含有 9 个不同的实验模块，如图 2 - 5 所示。实验者根据需要从中选择一个实验模块。当选择了一个实验模块之后，系统将自动设置该实验所需的各项参数，并且自动启动数据采样，直接进入实验状态。

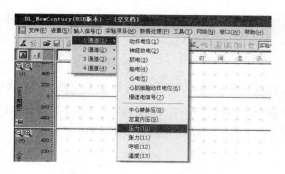

图 2-4 "输入信号"菜单
Fig. 2-4 "Input signal" menu

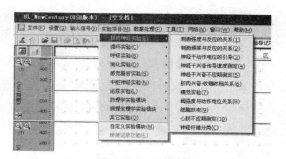

图 2-5 "实验项目"菜单
Fig. 2-5 "Experimental project" menu

4. 分时复用区　在 BL-420 软件主界面的最右边是一个分时复用区，包括：控制参数调节区（　按钮，调节增益、滤波、时间常数、扫描速度等），显示参数调节区（　按钮，调节各个通道显示参数，如前景色、背景色、格线色等），通用信息显示区（　按钮，显示各个通道测量的当前值、时间值、最大值、最小值、均值等数据），专用信息显示区（　按钮，显示实验模块专用的测量数据）。

在控制参数调节区，　增益调节旋钮用于调节通道增益，可使观察的信号图形增大或变小；　时间常数调节旋钮可用于衰减生物信号中所带入的低频噪声，而让高频信号通过；　滤波调节旋钮可用于衰减生物信号中带入的高频噪声，而让低频信号通过；　扫描速度按钮，可根据记录信号变化的快慢调节显示波形的扫描速度。

5. 其他常用工具按钮　　数据记录按钮，　开始按钮，　暂停按钮，　停止按钮，　通用实验标记按钮，　打开特殊实验标记对话框按钮。

四、BL-420 生物机能实验系统的使用

（一）启动软件
双击 WinXP 操作系统桌面上的"BL-420 软件"的快捷方式图标即可启动该软件。

（二）退出软件
选择 BL-420 软件"文件"菜单中的"退出"命令即可退出该软件。

（三）选定输入信号
有下述两种输入信号方法，选择其中任何一种方式均可开始记录生物信号：

1. 用菜单命令选择区中"输入信号"命令选定实验者自己确定的信号输入方式（自由组合），比如"1"通道选择"心电"，"2"通道选择"压力"，"3"通道选择"张力"。

2. 用菜单命令选择区中"实验项目"菜单中已确定好的实验模块，比如循环实验中的血流动力学模块等。一旦选定后，就有相应的参数设定对话框出现，根据实验要求设定所需参数，即可进行信号的采集、记录。

（四）刺激器参数设置
刺激器调节区包含两个与刺激器调节相关的按钮，分别是"打开刺激器设置对话框"按

7

钮（![按钮]，可以设置模式和刺激的方式、频率、强度等，如图 2 - 6 所示）和"启动/停止刺激"按钮（![按钮]）。

（五）添加通用实验标记或特殊实验标记

单击 ![按钮] 按钮可以添加通用实验标记，单击 ![按钮] 按钮可以打开特殊实验标记编辑对话框，如图 2 - 7 所示。可以在特殊实验标记编辑对话框中选择一个已经编辑好的特殊实验标记组，或者自己新建一个特殊实验标记组，然后按"确定"按钮选择该组特殊标记。

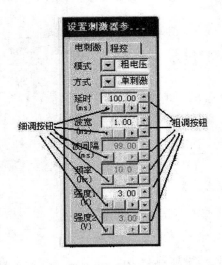

图 2 - 6　设置刺激器参数对话框

Fig. 2 - 6　**Dialog box of stimulation parameters configuration**

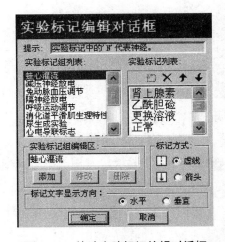

图 2 - 7　特殊实验标记编辑对话框

Fig. 2 - 7　**Dialog box of special experimental tag editor**

（王银环）

第二节　常用仪器的使用

一、电子天平（Electronic balance）

电子天平称量准确可靠、显示快速清晰，按照精度可分为以下几类：①超微量电子天平；②微量天平；③半微量天平；④常量电子天平；⑤分析天平；⑥精密电子天平。机能实验室常用的是半微量天平和常量电子天平，如图 2 - 8、图 2 - 9 所示。微量天平主要用于称量用量少的药品，如组胺、乙酰胆碱等。常量电子天平主要用于实验室老师配药和学生鼠类动物实验的称重等。使用时注意天平载重不得超过最大载荷，被称物品应放在干燥清洁的器皿中称量；称量完毕后，及时取出被称物品，并保持天平清洁。

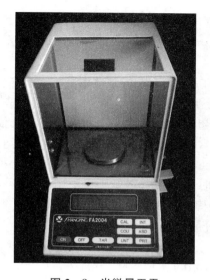

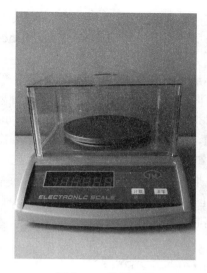

图 2 - 8　半微量天平

Fig. 2 - 8　Semi-micro balance

图 2 - 9　常量天平

Fig. 2 - 9　Constant balance

二、智能热板仪（Intelligent hot plate apparatus）

RB - 200 智能热板仪（图 2 - 10）采用液晶显示技术，提供轻触式按钮，实验数据可现场打印，也可与计算机连接，传送实验数据。在机能实验教学中，此仪器主要用于镇痛药物实验。使用时须注意开机后先加热到设定温度，系统默认是"55℃"，在达到设定温度前不要进行实验；配备的手动按钮，实验时才能使用，不能用于其他计时的工作，以免减少其使用寿命。

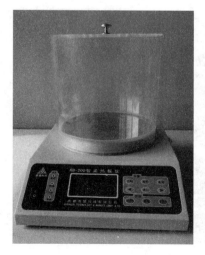

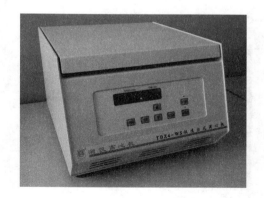

图 2 - 10　RB - 200 智能热板仪

Fig. 2 - 10　RB - 200 intelligent hot plate apparatus

图 2 - 11　TDZ4 - WS 低速离心机

Fig. 2 - 11　TDZ4 - WS conventional centrifuge

三、离心机 （Centrifugal machine）

离心是利用离心机转子高速旋转产生的强大的离心力，加快液体中颗粒的沉降速度，把样品中不同沉降系数和浮力密度的物质分离开。依据转速不同，离心机分为低速离心机（<6 000 r/min）、高速离心机（<25 000 r/min）和超速离心机（>30 000 r/min）；依据温度控制不同，离心机分为冷冻离心机和普通离心机，冷冻离心机带有制冷系统，能够控制温度最低至-20℃，普通离心机不带制冷系统。在机能实验教学中，常用的是低速离心机，用于药物半衰期的测定实验，如图2-11所示。使用时离心管一定要用天平平衡重量（重量平衡），盖上离心管盖子并旋紧；完成离心时，要等待离心机自动停止，不允许用手或其他物件迫使离心机停转，待转头完全静止后，才能打开舱门。

四、722S 分光光度计 （722S spectrophotometer）

722S型可见分光光度计在近紫外和可见光谱区域内对样品物质作定性和定量的分析，是理化实验室常用的分析仪器之一，如图2-12所示。在机能实验教学中，用于药物半衰期的测定实验。使用时，避免阳光直射、震动、尘埃和腐蚀性物质侵蚀；注意随时操作置0%（T）、100%（T），确保测试结果有效。

五、HW-400 恒温平滑肌槽 （Thermostat smooth muscle slot）

恒温平滑肌槽主要用于离体肠管平滑肌等实验中，调节和维持实验环境（如实验药液）温度，从而保证离体平滑肌的生理活性，使相关实验顺利进行，如图2-13所示。实验前需要开机加热10~20 min，确保肌槽内达到实验要求的温度（一般是37℃）；调节气量时，不要用力太大，以免损坏调节钮；实验结束时，一定要清洗大、小药筒，并将肌槽倒置控干，以免遗留液体腐蚀机器。

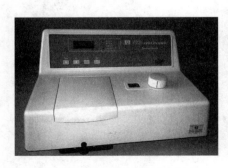

图 2-12　722S 分光光度计
Fig. 2-12　722S spectrophotometer

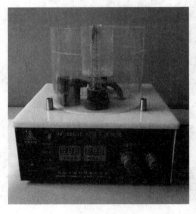

图 2-13　HW-400 恒温平滑肌槽
Fig. 2-13　HW-400 thermostat smooth muscle slot

（王建辉　耿　菲）

第三节　常用实验器材及手术器械

一、婴儿秤（Baby scale）

实验用家兔的大小与出生婴儿相当。婴儿秤由于其结构中有个大的托盘，所以也可用于家兔的称重。使用时禁止激烈震动，待动物身体平稳时再读数，以免影响称量值。

二、换能器（Transducer）

换能器是将能量从一种形式变成为另一种形式的器件。机能实验学常用的换能器有张力换能器和压力换能器两类，是分别将张力、压力机械信号转变为电信号，然后输入不同的仪器进行处理，以便对其所代表的生理变化作深入的分析。

（一）张力换能器（Tension transducer）

1. 原理与结构　张力换能器是利用某些导体或半导体材料在外力作用下发生变形时，其电阻会发生改变的"应变效应"原理。将由这些材料做成的应变片元件作为桥式电路的两对电阻，并与一个直流电源相接，当外力作用于换能器使其发生轻度弯曲时，由于电桥失去平衡，产生微弱的电流信号，可通过 BL－420 生物机能实验系统将其放大后输入微机显示（图 2－14）。

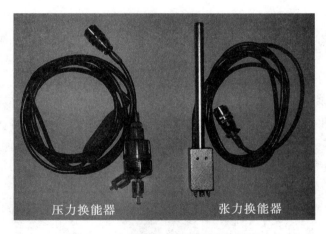

压力换能器　　　　张力换能器

图 2－14　张力换能器和压力换能器
Fig. 2－14　Tension transducer and pressure transducer

2. 使用方法与注意事项

（1）使用方法：使用时先将换能器固定在铁支架台上，一端与记录装置相连，另一端与被测对象相连，并使连接线保持适当的张力，开启记录仪，描记信号。

（2）注意事项：根据量程不同，张力换能器分为 0～10 g、0～50 g 和 0～100 g 等几种型号，根据所作实验选择适当量程的换能器，以免过负荷而损坏换能器；换能器要水平地安置在支架上，使用时不能用力牵拉或碰撞，以免损坏换能器；使用时，防止液体渗入换能器。

11

（二）压力换能器（Pressure transducer）

1. 原理与结构　原理同张力换能器。压力换能器头端是一个半球形的结构，其内面后部为薄片状的应变元件，组成桥式电路。其前端有两个短管开口，位于正中央的是压力输入口；位于侧壁的是排气口（图 2-14）。

2. 使用方法与注意事项

（1）使用方法：换能器在进行测量前，将压力输入口和排气口分别与三通接好，向压力换能器内注入抗凝溶液并排出换能器内的气泡，不得有泄漏现象。将换能器与大气相通以确定零压力基线。然后将换能器与充满抗凝液测压导管相通，即可进行压力测量。

（2）注意事项：使用时确保换能器和动脉插管内没有气泡；用完后应及时清除换能器内的液体或血液，晾干以备再用；压力换能器里有一个圆形橡胶圈，一定要垫好，冲洗换能器时不要遗失。

三、电　极（Electrode）

电刺激通过电极作用于组织或细胞，使其产生反应。最常用的电极依其使用目的不同，可分为普通电极、保护电极、锌铜弓等（图 2-15）。

（一）普通电极（Ordinary electrode）

通常是在一绝缘管的前端安装两根电阻很小的金属丝（常用银丝或不锈钢丝），金属丝后端各连有一条导线，可与刺激器的输出端相接。常用于记录神经干动作电位、骨骼肌肌电等。

（二）保护电极（Shielded electrode）

保护电极的特点是前端的银丝嵌在绝缘保护套中，使用此种电极刺激在体神经干时，可保护组织不受刺激。

（三）锌铜弓（Bimetal electrode）

锌铜弓是一个带有简单锌铜电池的双极刺激电极，常用来检查坐骨神经腓肠肌标本的功能状况。其结构是平行排列的一根粗锌丝和一根粗铜丝，两者顶端焊接在一起，当锌铜弓与湿润的活体组织接触时，由于 Zn 较 Cu 活泼，易失去电子形成正极，使细胞膜超极化，Cu 得到电子成为负极，使细胞膜去极化而兴奋。电流按从 Zn 端到活体组织、再到 Cu 端的方向流动。

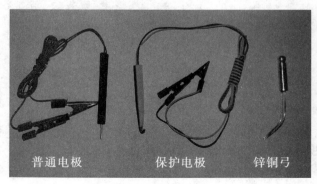

图 2-15　机能实验常用电极

Fig. 2-15　Electrodes commonly used in functional experiments

四、肌　槽（Muscle slot）

肌槽一般都装有两对刺激电极、一个安装标本的插孔及固定螺丝，侧方是一根用来固定肌槽的金属棍。安装标本时操作要轻，不要使标本受牵拉和被污染，以保持标本良好的兴奋性。先将神经搭在电极上，将肌肉附着的股骨插入电极旁的小孔内，拧紧固定螺丝，再将肌肉游离端结扎线与张力换能器悬梁臂前端的小孔中穿线的挂钩相连。然后，上下移动铁支架上固定张力换能器的双凹夹，使缚线刚处于拉直状态。

五、神经标本屏蔽盒（Shielding box for nerve specimen）

通常是用有机玻璃制成，盒内有两根导轨，导轨上有七根装有银丝电极的有机玻璃滑块，电极滑块可以在导轨上随意移动，用以调节电极间的距离。每个电极滑块通过导线与标本盒侧壁的一个接线相连，其中一对作为刺激电极，一对作为记录电极，记录电极与刺激电极间的电极接地。

使用时，先将标本盒用导线与 BL - 420 生物机能实验系统相连，将神经搭在刺激电极一侧，再将肌肉游离端结扎线与张力换能器悬梁臂前端的小孔中穿线的挂钩相连。然后，上下移动铁支架上固定张力换能器的双凹夹使缚线刚处于拉直状态。神经标本屏蔽盒常用于生理神经干动作电位实验。

六、缺氧瓶（Hypoxia bottle）

缺氧瓶用于缺氧实验中，分为兔缺氧瓶和鼠缺氧瓶两种。兔缺氧瓶用广口瓶装钠石灰，外接两根玻璃管，其中一根插乳胶管与气管插管相连，另外一根下缚气囊，与大气相通。鼠缺氧瓶也装有钠石灰，把小鼠直接放入缺氧瓶内，并与 CO 发生装置相连。

七、哺乳类动物常用手术器械（Surgical instruments for mammals）

（一）手术刀（Scalpel）
刀柄一端为一个良好的钝性分离器，可用以分离组织，或用以显露手术野深部。刀片宜用血管钳夹持安装，避免割伤手指。持刀方式有多种，如执弓式、执笔式、握持式、反挑式等。可根据手术切口的大小、深浅、精细程度及组织结构特点等情况而定。

（二）手术剪（Surgical scissors）
分直、弯两型，各型又分长、短两种，长型剪多用于深部手术，短型剪用于浅部手术。持剪的方法是以拇指和环指分别插入剪柄环，中指放在环指指环的前外方柄上，示指轻压在剪柄和剪刀片交界处的轴节处。手术剪适用于剪神经、血管、脂肪等组织，禁用其剪骨头等坚硬组织。

（三）止血钳（Hemostatic forceps）
根据大、小、直、弯形状可分为多种型号。用来夹闭出血点，分离和牵引组织等，但因其对组织有压轧作用，易造成组织损伤，所以不宜用其夹持皮肤、脏器及脆弱的组织。持钳

13

方法同手术剪。

（四）手术镊（Surgical forceps）

分有齿镊、无齿镊和眼科镊。有齿镊用于夹持皮肤，无齿镊用于夹持皮下组织、脂肪、黏膜等，细小的眼科镊适于分离血管、神经干或夹镊细小软组织。持镊时，用拇指对示指和中指，不宜握于掌心内，初学者应特别注意。

（五）眼科剪（Eye scissors）

常用来剪包膜、神经或剪破血管以便插管。禁用眼科剪剪皮肤、肌肉、骨骼等。使用方法同手术剪。

（六）持针器（Acutenaculum）

在缝合皮肤、肌肉、血管、神经等各种组织时用来夹持缝合针。使用时，用持针器的尖端夹住缝合针近尾端1/3处。执持针器时，仅用手掌握住其环部即可，不必将手指插入环口中。

（七）动脉夹（Arterial clip）

有大小之分。根据动脉的粗细或手术操作空间大小选用。用于夹闭动脉阻断血液流动，以便动脉插管。

（八）插管与导管（Cannula and catheter）

以玻璃管拉制成的"Y"和"卜"形气管插管有大小之分，可根据动物气管直径大小选择。急性动物实验时插入气管，以保持呼吸通畅。以粗细不同的塑料管和玻璃管制成的导管，可作动脉、静脉、淋巴管、输尿管插管。

部分哺乳动物手术器械如图2-16所示。

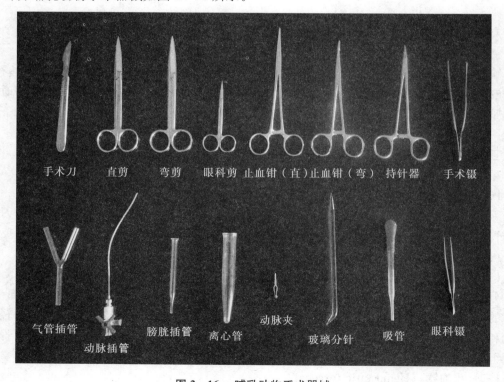

图 2 - 16　哺乳动物手术器械

Fig. 2 - 16　Surgical instruments for mammals

八、两栖类动物手术器械（Surgical instruments for amphibians）

（一）剪刀（Scissors）

普通粗剪用于剪皮肤、肌肉和骨骼等粗硬组织。眼科剪用于剪血管、神经、心外膜等细软组织，不能用于剪粗硬组织。

（二）金属探针（Metal probe）

用于破坏蛙类的脑和脊髓组织。

（三）镊子（Forceps）

大有齿镊用于剥脱蛙皮、夹捏肌肉和骨骼。眼科镊用于分离血管、神经或夹捏细小的软组织，不可直接夹捏或牵拉血管和神经。

（四）蛙手术板（Frog operation board）

由木板制成，用图钉或大头针将蛙肢体固定在蛙手术板上，便于解剖和实验。

（五）玻璃分针（Glass dissecting needle）

用于钝性分离血管和神经干的周围组织，暴露血管和神经干。

（六）蛙心夹（Frog heart clip）

用于夹住蛙心尖部位，夹尾孔穿线与张力换能器相连，以描记蛙心舒缩活动。

九、人体实验常用器材（Human experimentation instruments）

（一）血压计（Sphygmomanometer）

机能实验最常用的是台式水银血压计，由检压计、袖带、橡皮球三部分组成，详细结构和使用方法见相关章节。

使用血压计时应注意观察，使用前未加压时零位要在 4 mmHg；加压后，在不放气时，水银柱在 1 min 内下降不应超过 4 mmHg，加压时禁止有断柱或气泡出现，如有气泡，应停止加压进行检查维修。在测量过程中根据患者的脉搏跳动速率控制泄气速度，对心率慢者应尽量慢速。使用完毕将血压计右倾斜 45°，使水银收入水银壶中后，再关好水银壶开关。

（二）视野计（Perimeter）

弧形视野计是一种检查人眼周边视野的仪器，由弧架、手柄、底座及各色视标组成，详细结构和使用方法见相关章节。测定时选用适宜的视标，从圆弧周边向中心缓慢移动。嘱被检者刚一发现视标或辨出颜色时，立即告知。将此时视标在弧上的位置记录在周边视野图上。

（三）听诊器（Stethoscope）

主要由拾音部分（胸件），传导部分（胶管）及听音部分（耳件）组成。听诊器通常应用的体件有两种类型：一是钟型，适于听取低调声音；一是膜型，适于听取高调声音。机能实验中，常用以听取人和实验动物肺部的正常与病理呼吸音、心音。

（四）音叉（Tuning fork）

音叉是呈"Y"形的钢质或铝合金发声器，各种音叉可因其质量和叉臂长短、粗细不同而在振动时发出不同频率的纯音。音叉检查是鉴别耳聋性质（传音性聋或感音性聋）的常用诊查方法，具体操作见相关章节。

（王建辉　耿　菲）

第三章 常用实验动物与动物实验基本知识

第一节 实验动物的种类与选择

一、常用实验动物的种类及特点

(一) 青蛙和蟾蜍

青蛙和蟾蜍的心脏在离体情况下仍可有节律性搏动，可应用于心脏功能方面的实验研究。用蟾蜍后肢制作的坐骨神经-腓肠肌标本常用于神经肌肉的生理功能观察和药物试验。利用蛙下肢血管灌注方法可进行水肿和各种因素对血管作用的实验。此外，还可以用于肾功能不全等方面的实验。蟾蜍皮肤粗糙，背部皮肤上有许多疣状突起的毒腺，分泌蟾酥，实验时注意不要溅入眼内，一旦进入眼内要及时用自来水冲洗。

(二) 小鼠

小鼠食管细长，约 2 cm，胃容量小（1.0～1.5 ml），不耐饥饿，对疾病的抵抗力差。雄性小鼠可见阴囊内睾丸下垂，外生殖器与肛门之间的距离长，两者间有毛生长；雌性小鼠外生殖器与肛门间距离短，两者之间无毛，可见到一条纵行的沟，成熟雌鼠的腹部可见乳头。广泛应用于各种药物的毒理实验、药物筛选实验、肿瘤研究实验、营养学实验、遗传学实验、内分泌、免疫、缺氧、水肿及其他多种疾病的实验研究。

(三) 大鼠

大鼠性情较凶猛、抗病力强。大鼠门齿较长，抓捕时易咬人。大鼠无胆囊且不能呕吐，不适宜用于任何有关呕吐的实验研究。常用品种为 Wistar 大鼠和 Sprague Dawley（SD）大鼠。常用于水肿、休克、炎症、心功能不全等各类实验。

(四) 豚鼠

豚鼠又名荷兰猪，其习性温顺，胆小易惊。其嗅觉、听觉较发达，对各种刺激均有极高的反应。豚鼠回肠自发活动较少，多用于离体肠管实验。豚鼠也常用于钾代谢紊乱、酸碱代谢紊乱、肺水肿等实验研究。

(五) 兔

家兔性情温顺、胆小怕惊。家兔肺被肋胸膜和肺胸膜隔开，心脏又被心包胸膜隔开。因此，开胸后打开心包胸膜暴露心脏进行实验操作时，只要不弄破纵隔膜，动物不需要做人工呼吸。在机能实验学中常用于呼吸及血压的调节、钾代谢紊乱、水肿、缺氧、休克、心功能不全、肝性脑病等实验。

二、实验动物分类

（一）遗传学分类方法

1. **近交系动物**　指连续全同胞兄妹交配 20 代（或以上），近交系数达 98% 以上、群体基因达到高度纯合和稳定的动物群。常用的近交系动物有 BALB/c 小鼠、C57BL/6J 小鼠等。

2. **封闭群动物**　封闭群动物是一个长期与外界隔离，雌雄个体之间能够随机交配的动物群。通常把 5 年以上不从外部引种，只在群体内进行随机交配的动物群称为封闭群。常用的封闭群动物有昆明小鼠、新西兰白兔、Wistar 大鼠和 Sprague Dawley 大鼠等。

3. **突变系动物**　正常染色体的基因发生了突变，具有了各种遗传缺陷的品系。常用的突变系动物有肥胖症小鼠、糖尿病小鼠、白内障大鼠等。

4. **系统杂交动物**　两个不同近交系杂交所产生的第一代动物为系统杂交动物。系统杂交动物若进一步交配繁殖杂交二代动物，则会出现遗传分离和基因重组，个体间的一致性就会消失，因此系统杂交动物不能进一步繁殖而保持其遗传组成不变。

（二）微生物学分类方法

1. **普通动物**　饲养在开放环境中，未经积极的微生物控制，不携带主要人畜共患病和动物烈性传染病病原体的动物称之为普通动物。一般可用于实验教学中的急性动物实验，不适用于科学研究。

2. **清洁动物**　是指除普通动物应排除的病原体外，不携带对动物危害大和对科学研究干扰大的病原体动物。清洁动物比普通动物健康，在一般的科学实验中被广泛应用。

3. **无特定病原体动物**　是指除上述两种动物应排除的病原体外，不携带主要潜在感染或条件致病菌和对科学实验干扰大的病原体的实验动物。多适用于长期慢性实验，实验结果相对可靠。

4. **无菌动物**　是指通过无菌剖宫产并在绝对屏障系统中饲养的动物，此种动物用现有的检测技术手段能够证明不携带任何微生物和寄生虫。

5. **悉生动物**　是指动物体内携带某种或某几种已知微生物或寄生虫，并在屏障系统内饲养的动物。悉生动物来源于无菌动物，通过接种一种或几种微生物而获得。

三、实验动物的选择

由于各种动物具有不同的特点，每一项科学研究都要求用适宜的实验动物，必须根据实验动物的特点及实验内容的需要来选择符合要求的动物。

（一）实验动物的选择原则

1. **近似性原则**　某些实验动物在组织结构、生理功能、群体分布、年龄状态和疾病特征等方面与人类有一定程度的相关性，如大型灵长类动物；或在某些组织器官的结构和功能上与人类近似，如狗的循环系统、神经系统和消化过程与人相似，猪的皮肤组织结构和功能上与人相似等。此外，在对某种疾病进行研究时，最好能找到与人类疾病相同的动物自发性疾病，或用动物复制的疾病模型尽可能近似人类疾病。

2. **差异性原则**　各种动物之间在基因型、组织型、代谢型、易感性等方面存在差异。

根据实验目的可选择具有特殊组织结构和生理功能的动物。如以呕吐为指标的实验研究一般选择狗和猫，而不用不易产生呕吐的草食动物如豚鼠等。

3. 易化原则　从易化的角度入手，应选择那些既能满足实验要求，结构、功能又简单，便于观察和分析的动物。如用蛙进行神经反射弧实验等。

4. 相容和匹配原则　实验所用的动物品质应与实验设计、实验条件、实验技术、实验仪器、设备等方面的水平相匹配，避免资源的浪费。

5. 可获性原则　具有饲养容易、繁殖周期短、多胎性、遗传和微生物控制方便等特点的动物，如大鼠、小鼠、兔等哺乳动物是医学实验研究中常用的动物。

6. 重复性和均一性原则　在实验研究中，应选用个体差异小，有很好的遗传均质性的动物，以保证实验结果的可重复性和均一性。

（二）实验动物的个体选择

1. 年龄、体重　一般而言，年幼动物较成年动物敏感，应根据实验目的不同而选用不同年龄的动物。急性实验多选用成年动物，慢性实验宜选用年轻一些的动物。动物的年龄可根据体重进行推算，大体上，成年小白鼠为 $20\sim30$ g；大白鼠为 $180\sim250$ g；豚鼠为 $450\sim700$ g；家兔为 $2.0\sim2.5$ kg。同一批次实验所选用动物年龄、体重应基本一致。

2. 性别　实验证明，性别不同的动物对相同致病因素的反应不同。例如，在心脏缺血再灌注损伤实验与氨基半乳糖实验性肝细胞性黄疸实验中，雄性大白鼠较雌性大白鼠容易成功。对性别无特殊要求的实验，宜选用雌雄各半。如已证明性别对实验无影响时，可雌雄不拘。

3. 生理状态　动物的特殊生理状态，如妊娠、哺乳等对实验结果影响很大，在选择实验动物时，应给予充分考虑。

4. 健康情况　实验证明，动物处于饥饿、寒冷、疾病等情况下，实验结果很不稳定。健康的动物表现为：发育良好，眼睛明亮，反应灵活，食欲良好，呼吸均匀，眼鼻部均无分泌物流出，皮毛清洁柔软而有光泽，腹部无隆起，肛门区清洁无稀便及分泌物，外生殖器无损伤、无脓痂及分泌物，爪趾无溃疡及结痂。

四、机能实验中对实验动物的保护

随着生命科学的不断发展，实验动物学及动物实验技术得到了长足发展。实验动物在基础医学教育特别是机能实验教学中应用极为广泛。作为研究者，应该通过科学、高效、经济的方法和人道主义原则不断改进和提高研究方法和质量，采取有效措施，使实验动物免遭不必要的伤害、惊恐、折磨、不适和疼痛，尽量减少实验动物的痛苦，维护实验动物的福利。在实验过程中，我们应该做到：

1. 善待实验动物，不随意使动物痛苦，尽量减少刺激强度和缩短实验时间。

2. 实验过程中应给予动物镇静、麻醉，以减轻和消除动物的痛苦；对于可能引起动物痛苦和危害的实验操作，应小心进行，不得粗暴。

3. 对于清醒的实验动物应进行一定的安抚，以减轻它们的恐惧和不良反应。

4. 实验外科手术过程中应积极落实实验动物的急救措施，对于术后或需要淘汰的实验动物要实施"安乐死"。

实验动物是生命科学研究不可缺少的支撑条件，是为人类的健康和发展作出贡献和牺牲的生命体。爱护动物、善待动物是人类的责任，是人类文明道德的需要，也是人与自然和谐发展的需要。

（朱丽艳）

第二节　动物实验基本知识

一、实验动物的编号、捉拿与固定

（一）实验动物的编号

实验时应将动物进行标记以示区分，通常根据实验动物的种类、数量以及实验时间的长短等选择编号方法，常用的实验动物编号方法有以下几种：

1. 染色法　染色法是指使用化学药品在实验动物身体的明显部位染色。常用的染色化学药品为 3‰～5‰ 苦味酸溶液，可将动物染成黄色。该方法对于实验周期短的实验动物较为合适，时间较长容易掉色。染色时动物取俯卧位，左前肢为 1；左后肢为 2；右后肢为 3；右前肢为 4；头部为 5；尾部为 10；背部为 20。

2. 挂牌法　挂牌法是将号码烙印在金属牌上，挂在实验动物的颈部、耳部、肢体或笼具上，用来区别实验动物的一种方法。该方法适用于狗等大型动物。

3. 烙印法　烙印法是用刺数钳（又称耳号钳）将号码打在动物耳朵上的一种编号方法。编号前先用酒精棉球将耳朵擦净，用刺数钳刺上号码，之后在烙印部位用棉球涂抹溶在食醋里的黑墨水。该法适用于耳朵比较大的动物，如家兔、狗等。

4. 打孔法　打孔法是用打孔机在实验动物的耳朵上打孔的编号方法，根据打在动物耳朵上的部位和孔的多少，来区分实验动物。打孔后必须用消毒过的滑石粉抹在打孔局部，以免耳孔闭合。

（二）实验动物的捉拿与固定

1. 小鼠　用右手捉住小鼠尾部，将其提起放在笼盖或表面粗糙的物体上，向后轻拉鼠尾，当小鼠向前爬行时，用左手拇指和示指捏住其两耳和颈部皮肤，手掌心、环指和小指夹住小鼠的背部皮肤和尾部，如图 3-1 所示。这类捉拿方法多用于灌胃、肌内注射、腹腔注射和皮下注射等。某些实验还需要固定小鼠。一般将小鼠呈仰卧位（必要时先进行麻醉）置于实验板上，用橡皮筋或棉线固定其四肢。在一些特殊的实验中，如尾静脉注射时，还需要使用特殊的固定装置进行固定。

2. 大鼠　大鼠受到惊吓或被激怒时容易咬伤操作者，捉拿大鼠时操作者应戴上防护手套（如帆布手套），右手轻轻抓住大鼠尾部向后拉，注意不要抓其尾部尖端，以防止尾巴尖端皮肤脱落，左手拇指和示指捏住其双耳和颈部皮肤，其余三指抓住其背部皮肤。大鼠的固定方法与小鼠相似，除固定四肢外，还应将其门齿固定，以防咬伤。

3. 家兔　家兔比较温顺，不咬人，但其脚爪较尖，捉拿时应避免被其抓伤。捉拿时先轻轻打开笼门，不要使其受惊。一只手抓住家兔的颈部皮毛将其提起，另一只手托住家兔的臀部，如图 3-2 所示。将家兔放在实验台上，即可进行采血、注射等实验操作。固定家兔的方法有台式固定和盒式固定。台式固定适用于测量血压、呼吸和进行手术操作等，固定时

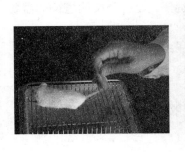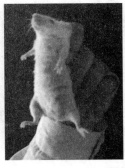

图 3-1　小鼠的捉拿

Fig. 3-1　Handling of a mouse

将其四肢拉直用绳绑在兔台四周的固定木块上，头部用一根粗棉绳将其门齿绑在兔台铁柱上。盒式固定适用于采血和耳缘静脉注射等。

　　4. 豚鼠　豚鼠胆小易受惊吓，抓取时必须稳、准、迅速。先用手掌迅速扣住豚鼠背部，抓住其肩胛上方，用拇指和示指环握其颈部，另一只手托住其臀部。豚鼠的固定方法与大鼠相同。

　　5. 蟾蜍　蟾蜍皮肤湿滑不易抓取，捉拿时可先在其体部包一层湿布，用左手将其背部贴紧手掌固定，拉直后肢，并用左手的中指、环指及小指夹住前肢，头部用拇指和示指压住，右手即可进行实验操作。抓取蟾蜍时注意不要挤压两侧耳部突起的毒腺，以免蟾蜍将毒液射到操作者的眼睛里。需要长时间固定时，可将蟾蜍麻醉或毁脑脊髓，再用大头针钉在蛙板上。

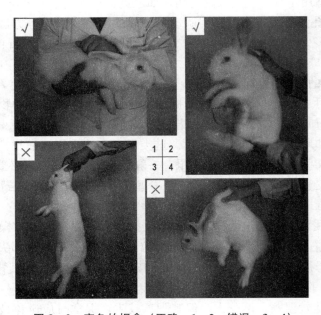

图 3-2　家兔的捉拿（正确：1、2；错误：3、4）

Fig. 3-2　Handling of a rabbit（1 and 2 are right；3 and 4 are wrong）

二、实验动物的给药途径与方法

（一）注射给药

1. **皮下注射** 用左手拇指和示指提起动物的皮肤，右手将注射器刺入皮下即可注射，拔针时针孔轻按片刻，以防药液漏出。不同实验动物皮下注射的部位不同，小鼠在背部或前肢腋下，大鼠在背部或侧下腹部，豚鼠在后大腿内侧或小腹部，家兔在背部或耳根。小鼠皮下注射如图3-3所示。

2. **腹腔注射** 实验对象为大鼠、小鼠时，用左手抓住动物使其腹部向上，并使头部处于低位，右手将注射器针头于左（或右）下腹部刺入皮下，将针头向前推0.5～1.0 cm，再以45°角穿过腹肌，此时有落空感，回抽无肠液、尿液、血液，即可注入药液。小鼠腹腔注射如图3-4所示。小鼠、大鼠腹腔注射剂量分别为0.1～0.2 ml/10 g和0.5～1.0 ml/100 g。若实验动物为家兔，进针部位为下腹部的腹白线旁1 cm处。

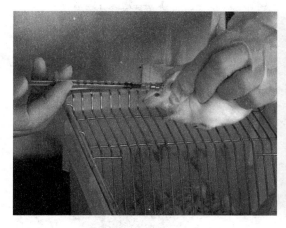

图3-3　小鼠皮下注射
Fig. 3-3　Subcutaneous injection of a mouse

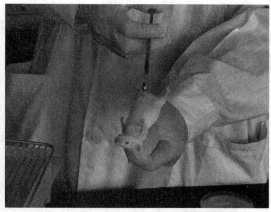

图3-4　小鼠腹腔注射
Fig. 3-4　Intraperitoneal injection of a mouse

3. **肌内注射** 注射应选肌肉发达且无大血管通过的部位，一般多选臀部。注射时垂直迅速刺入肌肉，回抽无回血即可注射。小鼠、大鼠等小动物肌内注射部位为大腿外侧肌肉。小鼠肌内注射如图3-5所示。

4. **静脉注射** 家兔选择耳外缘静脉注射，如图3-6所示。先拔去注射部位的被毛，用手指弹动或轻揉兔耳，或用乙醇擦拭，使静脉充盈，左手示指和中指夹住静脉的近心端，拇指绷紧静脉的远心端，环指和小指垫在下面，右手持注射器尽量从静脉的远端刺入，移动拇指于针头上加以固定针头，放开示指和中指，感觉顺畅或血管变白，即将药液注入，拔出针头后用手压迫针眼片刻。

小鼠和大鼠采用尾静脉注射，如图3-7和图3-8所示。鼠尾静脉共3根，左右两侧和背侧各1根，通常选两侧静脉注射。首先将动物固定在暴露尾部的固定器内，用75%乙醇反复擦拭鼠尾使血管扩张，并使表皮角质软化，左手拇指及示指捏住鼠尾两侧使静脉充盈，注射时针头与尾部平行进针。先缓慢注入少量药液，如无阻力，表示针头已进入静脉，则可继续注入。注射完毕后把鼠尾向注射侧弯曲以止血。如需多次注射，应尽可能从末端开始，以后向尾根部方向移动注射。

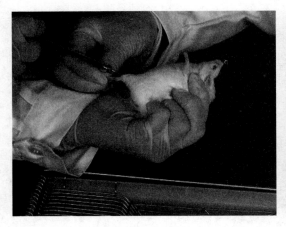 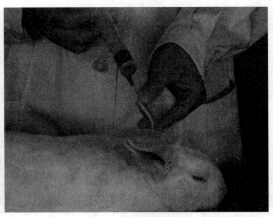

图 3 - 5　小鼠肌内注射
Fig. 3 - 5　Intramuscular injection of a mouse

图 3 - 6　家兔耳缘静脉注射
Fig. 3 - 6　Ear vein injection of a rabbit

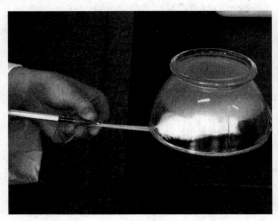 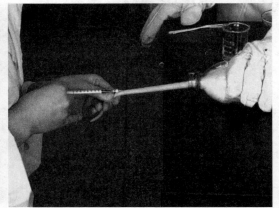

图 3 - 7　小鼠尾静脉注射
Fig. 3 - 7　Tail vein injection of a mouse

图 3 - 8　大鼠尾静脉注射
Fig. 3 - 8　Tail vein injection of a rat

（二）经口给药

小鼠、大鼠灌胃法　灌胃法是用灌胃器将药液灌到动物胃内。灌胃器由注射器和特殊的灌胃针构成。左手抓住鼠背部及颈部皮肤将动物固定成垂直体位，右手持灌胃器轻轻压其头部，使口腔与食管成一条直线，将灌胃针从动物嘴角插入其口中，沿上腭缓慢通过食管插入胃内，如动物没有挣扎则将可药液灌入；如果动物挣扎或遇阻力，则将灌胃针拔出重新灌胃。一般当灌胃针插入小鼠 3～4 cm，大鼠或豚鼠 4～6 cm 后可将药物注入。常用的灌胃量小鼠为 0.1～0.2 ml/10 g，最多不超过 1 ml；大鼠 0.5～1.0 ml/100 g。小鼠和大鼠灌胃方法如图 3-9 和图 3-10 所示。

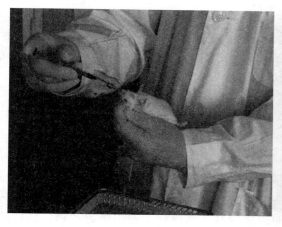

图 3－9　小鼠灌胃

Fig. 3－9　Gastric lavage of a mouse

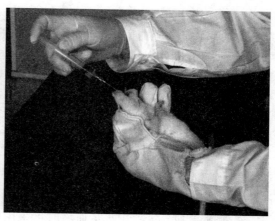

图 3－10　大鼠灌胃

Fig. 3－10　Gastric lavage of a rat

三、实验动物的麻醉方法

（一）全身麻醉

麻醉药经呼吸道吸入或静脉、肌内注射，抑制中枢神经系统，产生神志消失、全身不感疼痛、肌肉松弛和反射抑制等作用，这种方法称全身麻醉。

1. 吸入麻醉法　该法常用乙醚作麻醉药，用几个棉球浸润乙醚，迅速转入钟罩或箱内让其挥发，然后将动物投入，待其出现麻醉特征后取出，即可进行实验。实验过程中应随时观察动物的变化，必要时可将乙醚烧杯放在其鼻部，以维持麻醉的时间与深度。

2. 注射麻醉法　该法操作简便，是实验室最常采用的方法之一，常用的麻醉药有戊巴比妥钠、硫喷妥钠、氨基甲酸乙酯（乌拉坦）等。小鼠、大鼠和豚鼠常用腹腔注射进行麻醉，兔、狗等较大动物多静脉注射进行麻醉。注射麻醉药时，先用药量的 2/3，密切观察动物生命体征的变化，若已达到所需的麻醉程度，就不再注射剩下的麻醉药，避免麻醉过深抑制延髓呼吸中枢而导致动物死亡。常用的注射麻醉药的给药剂量及给药途径见下表。

常用麻醉药的剂量和给药途径

Administration of doses and routes commonly used anesthetics

麻醉药（常用浓度） Anesthetic	实验动物 Animal	给药途径 Route	给药剂量（mg/kg） Dose
戊巴比妥钠（3%～5%） Pentobarbital sodium	家兔 Rabbit 小鼠、大鼠、豚鼠 Mouse, rat, guinea pig	静脉注射 iv 腹腔注射 ip	25～30 45～50
硫喷妥钠（5%） Penthiobarbital sodium	家兔 Rabbit 小鼠 Mouse 大鼠 Rat	静脉注射 iv 腹腔注射 ip 腹腔注射 ip	15～20 40 15～20
氨基甲酸乙酯（25%） Ethyl urethane	家兔 Rabbit 小鼠、大鼠 Mouse, rat	静脉注射 iv 皮下或肌内注射 sc, im	1000 1000～1500

（二）局部麻醉

用局部麻醉药阻滞周围神经末梢或神经干、神经节、神经丛的冲动传导，产生局部的麻醉区，称为局部麻醉。其特点是动物保持清醒，对重要器官功能的干扰轻微，麻醉并发症少，是一种比较安全的麻醉方法。适用于大、中型动物短时间内的实验。

四、实验动物的取血方法

（一）大鼠、小鼠

1. 尾部取血　需要很少量血液时采用尾部取血。固定动物，将鼠尾置于45℃热水中浸泡数分钟使血管扩张，擦干鼠尾，剪去尾尖，从尾根部向尾尖部按摩，血即从尾尖流出。

2. 眼部取血　需要中等量血液时可采用眼球后静脉丛取血法。左手固定动物，轻轻压迫颈部两侧，使眼球充分外突，球后静脉丛充血。右手持毛细管将其插入内眦部，向眼底方向旋转插入，血液自行顺毛细管流出。

3. 大血管取血　可从颈动、静脉，股动、静脉，以及腹主动脉取血。将动物麻醉后固定，分离动、静脉，使其充分暴露，用注射器沿大血管平行方向刺入，抽取所需血量。

4. 心脏取血　将动物仰卧固定，心前区域去毛消毒，左手示指在左侧第3～4肋间摸到心尖搏动最强处，右手持连有针头的注射器在此穿刺。血液因心脏的跳动自行进入注射器。

5. 断头取血　左手抓住动物使其头部略低，右手用力剪断其颈部，血即可滴入容器。此方法用于实验结束后采集大量血液。

（二）家兔

1. 耳部取血

（1）耳缘静脉取血：固定家兔，取血部位去毛，轻揉兔耳使血管扩张，用粗针头刺破耳缘静脉，血液即可流出，取血后用棉球压迫止血。或者用注射器插入血管取血。

（2）耳中央动脉取血：固定家兔，取血部位去毛，轻揉兔耳使血管扩张，用注射器在中央动脉末端向心脏方向刺入血管，即可抽出血液。

2. 心脏取血　家兔仰卧固定，心脏部位去毛消毒，注射器刺入心尖搏动最强处，血液随即进入注射器。

五、实验动物的处死方法

（一）大鼠、小鼠的处死

1. 脊椎脱臼法　左手拇指和示指用力向下按住鼠头，右手抓住尾根部用力拉向后上方，鼠脊椎脱臼，使脊髓与脑髓拉断，动物立即死亡。

2. 断头法　用剪刀剪断鼠颈部，动物即可死亡。

3. 击打法　右手提起鼠尾，用力摔击其头部致死，或用木槌打击头部致死。

4. 二氧化碳吸入法　将动物置于木箱或塑料袋中，充入CO_2，几分钟后动物便死亡。

（二）家兔、豚鼠、狗的处死

1. 空气栓塞法　用注射器向动物静脉内注入一定量的空气，使之发生栓塞而死。一般兔和猫注入10～20 ml空气，狗注入70～150 ml空气。

2. 急性失血法　豚鼠可用注射器在心脏采集大量血液致死。狗等较大动物应先麻醉，之后暴露股三角区并作一个约 10 cm 的横切口，把股动、静脉全部切断，用湿纱布不断擦去股动脉切口周围处的血液和血凝块，同时不断用自来水冲洗流血，使切口处保持畅通，动物 3～5 min 内即可死亡。

3. 注射麻醉法　注射戊巴比妥钠致死。豚鼠用 3 倍以上麻醉剂量腹腔注射，猫用麻醉剂量的 2～3 倍剂量静脉或腹腔注射，家兔 80～100 mg/kg 耳缘静脉注射，狗 100 mg/kg 静脉注射。

（安春娜　薛　涛）

Section 2　Fundamentals of animal experimentation

1. Numbering, handling and restraint of experimental animals

（1）Numbering of experimental animals

Experimental animals should be marked so as to distinguish one from another. The commonly used means of animal identification are described as follow:

① Staining method　Chemicals are used to stain the obvious parts of the experimental animal's body. The commonly used staining chemical is 3%- 5% picric acid solution, which can dye the animal's body part to yellow. This method is more appropriate for the animals with a short experimental period, as the colour will fade over a long period of time. When staining, the animal should be restrained in the prone position; staining of the left forelimb indicates No. 1, left hindlimb is No. 2, right hindlimb is No. 3, right forelimb is No. 4, head is No. 5, tail is No. 10, and staining of the back is No. 20.

② Plaque method　A metal plate with an imprinted number can be hung on the experimental animal's neck, ears, limbs or on the cage. This method is suitable for the larger animals such as dogs.

③ Branding method　Pricking pliers (also known as ear marking pliers) is used to prick numbers on the ears of animals. The ear needs to be cleaned with alcohol wipes before it is pricked by the pliers; then the branded area is swabbed with black ink dissolved in vinegar. This method is suitable for the animals with larger ears, such as rabbits and dogs.

④ Hole punching method　A puncher is used to perforate holes in the ears of experimental animals for the purpose of encoding. The experimental animals are indentified based on the site and number of the holes. Sterilized talc must then be rubbed in the hole punched sites to avoid closure of the ear holes.

（2）Handling and restraint of experimental animals

① Mouse　The mouse is grasped by its tail with the right hand and placed on the cage lid or other rough surface. As its tail is pulled back gently, it is pinched by the scruff of the neck behind the ears with the left thumb and index finger while the mouse is crawling forward; meanwhile, its dorsal skin and the tail are gripped with the palm, ring finger and little finger (Fig. 3-1). This method is usually used for intragastric administration, intramuscular injection, intraperitoneal injection and subcutaneous injection. In some experiments where the mouse needs to be fixed, the mouse is placed on an experimental board in the supine position (anesthetized first when necessary) with its limbs restrained by rubber bands or cotton threads. In some special experiments, for example, when tail intravenous injection is involved, a specific fixing device may be applied in order to restrain the animal.

② Rat   Rats may try typically to bite the operator when they are frightened or agitated, so the operator should wear protective gloves when catching a rat. The rat tail is pulled backward with your right hand, but be sure not to catch the tip to prevent exfoliation of the tail tip skin. Then the scruff of the neck behind with the left thumb and index finger hold the dorsal skin with the remaining three fingers. Fixing of rats is similar with that of mice; besides the restraint of limbs, the incisor teeth should also be fixed to prevent being bitten.

③ Rabbit   Rabbits are docile and they usually don't bite, but their claws are sharp. Operators shall be cautious not to be scratched while catching rabbits. The cage gate shall be opened quietly to avoid frightening the rabbits. The operator should grasp the rabbit by the skin on the nape of the neck and lift it with one hand, and support the rump with the other hand (Fig. 3 – 2). After it is placed on the experimental table, the experimental procedures such as drawing blood and injection can then be preformed. Restraining of the rabbit includes tabletop fixation and box fixation. The tabletop fixation is suitable for blood pressure measurement, respiration measurement and surgical operations. Its four limbs are stretched and tied to the wooden blocks secured to the rabbit table, and the head is bound to the table by a thick rope around its incisors. Box style fixation is suitable for blood drawing or marginal ear vein injection.

④ Guinea pig   Guinea pigs are easily frightened, so handling must be performed in a steady, accurate and rapid manner. The handler should put the palm quickly on the back of the guinea pig, grasp it by the superior of the shoulders with the thumb and index finger around its neck, and hold the haunch with the other hand. Fixing methods for guinea pigs are the same as that for rats.

⑤ Toad   The skin of toads is damp and slippery and not easy to grasp. Handlers can wrap a layer of wet cloth around its body and restrain it by firmly holding the back of toad with the left palm. Its hindlimbs are then straightened. The forelimbs are clamped with the middle finger, ring finger and little finger of the left hand, and the head are pressed with the thumb and index finger, as shown in Fig. 4 – 1. Then the handler can conduct the experiment with his or her right hand. Do not squeeze the prominent venom glands located behind both ears to avoid toad venom being ejected into the eyes. If the experiment requires the toad to be restrained for a rather long time, the operator can anesthetize the toad or damage its spinal cord before fixing the toad onto a frog plate with pins.

2. Routes of administration for experimental animals

(1) Administration by injection

① Subcutaneous injection (sc)   After the skin is lifted with the left thumb and index finger, the syringe is inserted subcutaneously to make the injection with the right hand. Pressure should be applied to the injection site for a moment when the needle is withdrawn to prevent liquid leakage. The subcutaneous injection sites vary between different experimental animals, which are usually selected at the back or the forelimb armpit for mice, the back or the side of lower abdomen for rats, inner side of hind limbs or lower abdomen for guinea pigs, and the back or ear root for rabbits. Subcutaneous injection for mice is illustrated in Fig. 3 - 3.

② Intraperitoneal injection (ip)   When rats and mice are given intraperitoneal injection, hold the animal should be held with the left hand, leaving its abdomen upward and its head in a lower position. The springe needle is then inserted into subcutaneous tissue from its left or right hypogastric zone with the right hand; the needle is pushed forward for 0.5 - 1.0 cm and penetrates through the abdominal muscles at 45 degree angle. The drug solution is injected if is no intestinal juice or urine is aspirated. Intraperitoneal injection for mice is illustrated in Fig. 3 - 4. Intraperitoneal injection dosage for mice and rats are 0.1 - 0.2 ml/10 g and 0.5 - 1.0 ml/100 g, respectively. For rabbits, the injection site is 1 cm away from the linea alba abdominis of its hypogastric zone.

③ Intramuscular injection (im)   Most common intramuscular sites are muscular areas that do not have great vessels running through them, such as the haunch. The needle should be inserted into the muscle vertically and rapidly and if aspiration shows no blood then the injection can be made. For the smaller animals such as mice and rats, the injection site is lateral thigh muscles. Intramuscular injection for mice is illustrated in Fig. 3 - 5.

④ Intravenous injection (iv)   Rabbits receive intravenous injection through their marginal ear veins (Fig. 3 - 6). The operator should firstly locate the injection site and remove the hair. The ear needs to be tapped or gently stroked, or rubbed with alcohol to engorge the vein. The proximal part of the vein is clamped with the left index finger and middle finger, the distal end straightened with the thumb, and the ring finger and little finger are put under the ear as padding. The needle is inserted distally into the vein with the right hand; the thumb is used to apply pressure against the needle to immobilize it, the index finger and middle finger are then released to inject the drug solution when it feels smooth or the vein appears transparent. Pressure should be applied at the injection site upon the removal of needle.

The injection for mice and rats is always via caudal veins (Fig. 3 - 7 and Fig. 3 - 8). They have three caudal veins which respectively locate at left and right sides and dorsal part. We usually choose the left or right side vein for intravenous injection. The animal should firstly be put in a restrainer with its tail exposed. The tail is then wiped repeatedly with 75%

alcohol to dilate the vein and soften the keratin. The two sides of the tail should be pinched with the left thumb and index finger to engorge the vein, and the needle should be pushed forward in the parallel direction to the tail. A small amount of drug is initially injected slowly and injection can be continued if there is no resistance. Bend the tail towards the injection direction to stop bleeding upon completion. If multiple injections are involved, the injection should be started from the tail end so that other injections can be moved forward along the tail.

(2) Intragastric administration via mouth

Gastric lavage for mice and rats   This approach is to administer drugs into animal stomach by gastric lavage devices. Gastric lavage device consists of a syringe and a special gavage needle. The animal is restrained in a vertical position with the left hand holding its back and neck skin. Its head is gently pressed to make the mouth and esophagus in a straight line with the right hand that is also holding the gastric lavage device. The lavage needle is inserted into the mouth from the angulus oris and advanced into the stomach down along the palate and then the drug is poured in if the animal does not struggle. If there is resistance or the animal struggles, pull the lavage needle out and repeat the procedure again. Generally speaking, the injection can be made when the needle is inserted 3 – 4 cm for mice, or 4 – 6 cm for rats or guinea pigs. Commonly administered intragastric volume is 0.1 – 0.2 ml/10 g for mice, not exceeding 1 ml; 0.5 – 1.0 ml /100 g for rats. The intragastric administration for mice and rats are shown in Fig. 3 – 9 and Fig. 3 – 10.

(An Chunna)

第三节　家兔实验基本操作技术

在实验中，组织实施动物的手术方法是必须熟练掌握的一项基本实验学技术。本节介绍家兔急性实验中较为常用的一些基本手术技能，如家兔麻醉、气管插管、神经分离及动脉插管技术等，为后续生理调节、基本模型复制、药理作用等实验奠定基础。

一、麻醉与固定

在整体动物实验中，为了避免动物挣扎而影响实验结果，必须用麻醉药将动物麻醉后再进行实验，对保证实验的顺利进行有十分重要的作用。

1. 捉拿、称重　用右手抓住颈背部被毛与皮（此处皮较厚）将其提起，然后用左手托住其臀部，使兔身的重量大部分落于左手上，将家兔放置婴儿秤上称重。

2. 麻醉　注射器抽取25％氨基甲酸乙酯（又名乌拉坦），用量为1 g/kg，排空气泡。选择家兔外侧耳缘静脉注射给药。注射前先拔去耳缘部被毛，用手指轻弹兔耳，使静脉充盈。然后用左手示指与中指夹住静脉的近心端，阻止静脉血回流，用拇指和环指固定耳缘静脉远心端，右手持注射器从耳缘静脉远端开始进针，并顺血管平行方向深入1 cm，注射器进入血管后回抽，若有血或少量推注药液血管发白，即可注入药物。若一次穿刺不成功可由远及近再次穿刺，如图3－6所示。

麻醉深浅依据角膜反射、肌张力、对疼痛刺激的反应和呼吸进行判断。若角膜反射迟钝或消失，肌肉松弛，呼吸减慢，痛反应消失，表明药物已足量。手术过程中，如动物苏醒，需要继续麻醉时，可再经静脉缓慢注入总剂量的 1/5，以维持麻醉深度。

3. 固定　将家兔麻醉后，仰卧位固定于兔手术台。

二、颈部手术

（一）气管插管术

家兔急性实验中，为了保持动物呼吸道的畅通，一般先切开气管，插入气管插管，防止分泌物堵塞气道，然后再进行其他的手术操作。

1. 颈部剪毛，紧贴动物颈部皮肤，小心地剪去动物毛发。沿颈部正中在喉头与胸骨之间作 5～7 cm 的切口。

2. 止血钳钝性分离皮下结缔组织、颈部肌群，暴露气管。气管位于颈部正中，全部被胸骨舌骨肌与胸骨甲状肌所覆盖。用止血钳分开左右胸骨舌骨肌，在正中线沿其中缝插入并向头尾两端扩张创口。注意止血钳不能插入过深，以免损伤气管或其他小血管。也可采用两示指沿左右胸骨舌骨肌中缝轻轻向上下拉开，将左右胸骨舌骨肌向两侧拉开，即可见到气管。

3. 在喉头以下（甲状软骨下 0.5～1 cm 处）气管处，分离一段气管并穿线备用，于两个软骨环之间，向头端做"⊥"形切口。

4. 将适当口径的气管插管由切口向胸端插入气管内，用线结扎，再在插管的侧管上打结，以防插管滑出。插入后要检查管内有无血液，若有血液，须拔出插管经止血处理后再插入。

（二）颈部神经、血管分离术

颈总动脉位于气管外侧，其腹面被胸骨舌骨肌和胸骨甲状肌所覆盖，分离两条肌肉之间的结缔组织，在肌腱下可找到一条深红色较粗大的血管，用手触之有搏动感，此即为颈总动脉。颈总动脉与颈部神经被结缔组织膜束在一起，称颈部血管神经束，共同走行于颈动脉鞘内。根据各条神经的形态、位置和走向等特点来辨认，迷走神经最粗，外观最白，位于颈总动脉外侧，易于识别；交感神经比迷走神经细，位于颈总动脉的内侧，呈浅灰色；降压神经最细，位于迷走神经和交感神经之间，在家兔为一独立的神经，沿交感神经外侧走行，如图 3-11 所示。用左手拇指和示指捏起颈皮和颈肌，中指顶起外翻即可找到。右手用蚊式止血钳或玻璃分针，顺血管神经束内神经和血管的走行方向细心分离出颈总动脉及神经 2～3 cm 长即可，然后各穿手术线备用。分离原则为：先神经后血管，先细后粗。

颈外静脉位置较浅，位于颈部皮下。用左手拇指和示指捏住颈部左侧缘皮肤切口，其余三指从皮肤外向上顶起外翻，即可在胸锁乳突肌外缘处清晰见到粗而明显的颈外静脉。沿血管走向用玻璃分针钝性分离，暴露颈外静脉 3～5 cm，穿两根手术线备用。

（三）颈总动脉插管术

1. 动脉插管前耳缘静脉注射肝素生理盐水（1 000 U/kg）进行抗凝。

2. 手术线结扎左侧颈总动脉远心端，动脉夹夹住颈总动脉近心端。

3. 在远心端结扎线与动脉夹之间，用眼科剪在靠远心端结扎线的动脉上呈 45°角向心方向做一"V"形切口，切口不宜过大，约为管径的 1/3。

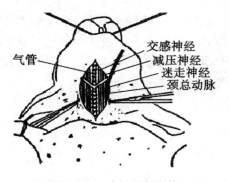

图 3-11　家兔颈部结构

Fig. 3-11　The cervical structure of rabbit

4. 将充满抗凝液的动脉插管向心方向插入动脉约 2 cm，结扎固定，并用远心端的结扎线围绕插管打结固定。

5. 打开动脉夹，动脉插管与压力换能器相连，通过 BL-420 生物机能实验系统监测血压。

（四）颈外静脉插管术

1. 用动脉夹夹闭颈外静脉的近心端。

2. 待血管内血液充分充盈后结扎颈外静脉的远心端。

3. 颈外静脉插管：用左手拇指与中指拉住远心端的结扎线，示指或小指从血管背后轻扶血管，右手持眼科剪向心方向呈 45°角，在靠远心端结扎线处作"V"形剪口，剪开血管直径约 1/3。

4. 将充满抗凝剂的静脉插管向心方向插入颈外静脉 2～3 cm，用已穿好的手术线扎紧插管，固定静脉插管防止滑脱，确认结扎固定牢靠后，放开动脉夹。

三、胸部手术

胸部正中剪毛，沿胸壁正中线胸锁关节处向下切开皮肤，开口 6～7 cm。分离左侧胸壁肌肉，如有出血，可用纱布压迫止血。找出左侧第 3、第 4 肋骨，用两把止血钳在靠近胸骨左缘处掰断左侧第 3、第 4 肋骨，开胸暴露心脏。

四、腹部手术

（一）膀胱插管术

腹部正中剪毛，耻骨联合向上沿腹正中切开皮肤约 5 cm。沿腹白线切开腹壁肌肉，将膀胱移至腹外。在膀胱顶部选择血管较少处做一荷包缝合，再在缝合线中心做一小切口，插入膀胱插管，收紧缝合线结扎固定，用小培养皿收集尿液。插管口最好正对着输尿管在膀胱的入口处，但不要紧贴膀胱后壁而堵塞输尿管。手术完毕后，用温热生理盐水纱布覆盖腹部切口。如果需要长时间收集尿样，则应关闭腹腔，如图 3-12 所示。

（二）十二指肠插管术

上腹部正中剪毛，从胸骨剑突下做 6～7 cm 上腹正中切口，打开腹腔。于上腹部找到

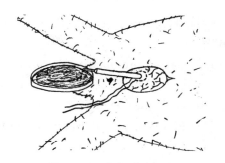

图 3 - 12　家兔膀胱插管

Fig. 3 - 12　Bladder cannulation of rabbit

胃，沿胃幽门向下找出十二指肠，肠系膜下穿线，在肠壁上剪一小口，将带有三通的细塑料插管向远端方向插入十二指肠内约 4 cm，用结扎线将肠管及插管系牢。将肠管回纳腹腔，用止血钳夹闭腹壁皮肤关闭腹腔，将三通插管尾端留置在外。

（张　娜　Daniel H. Nissen）

Section 3　Elementary operational techniques for rabbit experiments

In animal experiments, performing surgical operations is a fundamental experimental technique which students must learn to be skilled in. In this section, some fundamental operation skills commonly used in rabbit acute experiments are described. Now, to prepare for the following experiments, we discuss anesthesia methods for rabbits and fundamental operational techniques for rabbit experiments.

1. Animal anesthesia and restraint

The animal must be anesthetized prior to the operations for the whole animal experimentation. Anesthesia can relieve pain and keep the animal calm, so that the experiment can be conducted smoothly.

（1）Handling and weighing　To lift up a rabbit, the handler should grasp the loose skin around the rabbit's neck with the right hand and support the rabbit's rump with the left hand. It is wrong to hold the rabbit by its ears. The rabbit is then placed on a scale to measure its weight, based on which the dosage of anesthetic drugs to be administered is calculated.

（2）Anesthesia　The rabbit is anaesthetized with 25% ethyl carbamate (urethane) (1g/kg) by intravenous injection through its marginal ear vein. Firstly, a marginal ear vein is selected and the hair is removed. The ear is then gently tapped to make the vein more visible. Then the proximal of the marginal ear vein is clamped with the left index finger and middle finger to allow engorgement. With the distal of the marginal ear vein restrained by the thumb and the ring finger, the syringe needle should be inserted from the distal end of the marginal ear vein with the right hand and advanced about 1 cm along the vessel direction. Then the handler should aspirate to check the blood withdrawal or inject slowly and watch for clearing of the lumen. The position where we begin to inject anesthetic should be as near to the distal of the marginal ear vein as is possible, so that if a bulge occurs in the ear, the needle can be removed and the process can be repeated proximal to the previous site (Fig. 3 – 6).

Depth of anesthesia can be judged from corneal reflex, muscle tension, response to stimulus of pain and respiration. Proper drugged state is that respiration is deep, slow and steady, corneal reflex and responses to stimulus of pain disappear, and muscles are relaxed.

(3) Restraint the rabbit in the supine position onto the operating table after anesthesia.

2. Operation on neck

(1) Trachea intubation

① The hair of the rabbit neck should be sheared carefully, followed with a midline incision 5 – 7 cm in length from the larynx to the breastbone.

② The subcutaneous tissues are separated layer by layer with hands or hemostatic forceps to expose the trachea.

③ The operator should now separate the trachea 2 – 3 cm under the throat (do not touch the thyroid), pass a thread under it, and make a "⊥" shape incision on the trachea.

④ The tracheal cannula is inserted toward the chest direction and the cannula and the trachea are then tied together.

(2) Separation of nerves, carotid artery and external jugular vein

The common carotid artery is located at the lateral side of the trachea and covered by the neck muscles. It is pink and if we touch it with a finger, we can feel the pulse. The vagus is thick and the sympathetic nerve is thin, whereas the depressor nerve is the thinnest and often adheres to the sympathetic nerve. Generally, the depressor nerve is separated first, then the sympathetic nerve, the vagus, followed finally by the common carotid artery. A 2 – 3 cm in length of each nerve is separated from the surrounding tissues. Silk threads are put under each nerve and the carotid artery for further use. The left common carotid artery is used for artery intubation (Fig. 3 – 11).

The external jugular vein of rabbits is very wide and thick and easy to find. When you use your fingers to turn over the side of the skin incision, you can see a thick brown-purple blood vessel—the external jugular vein, on which you can not feel the pulse with your fingers. The external jugular vein should then be separated carefully along the vessel direction and the silk threads should be passed under it.

(3) Arterial cannulation

① Before the arterial cannula is inserted, 10^{-4} heparin should be injected through the marginal ear vein.

② At the distal end (as near as possible to the head), the left common carotid artery is ligated with a thread. Then the proximal end (as near as possible to the heart) is clamped with an arterial clip.

③ We use scissors to make an incision at the distal end between the ligation and the arterial clip (about 1/3 diameter of the artery) towards the heart, insert the arterial cannula into the artery at the incision and secure the top of the cannula with the silk thread; the side of cannula is ligated with the remaining thread to prevent the cannula turning around or the wall of the artery being cut by the top of the cannula. Keep the direction of the cannula along that of the vessel in order to avoid the cannula buckling.

(4) Venous cannulation

① Clamp the proximal vein with an artery clip.

② When the vein is fully engorged, ligate the distal end.

③ Make a "V" shape cut on the vein toward the heart, the size of which is about 1/3 of the vein diameter.

④ Insert the vein cannula 2 – 3 cm towards the heart direction. Then secure the vein cannula tightly in the vein with thread.

3. Operation on chest

(1) The animal is fixed in the supine position on the operating table after it has been anesthetized.

(2) The left chest wall muscles are separated and gauze compression hemostasis is applied to stop bleeding.

(3) The third and fourth ribs are located. Two hemostatic forceps are used near the left edge of sternum to break off the left third and fourth ribs. Then the chest is opened to expose the heart.

4. Operation on abdomen

(1) Bladder cannulation   The hair on the middle of the abdomen is sheared and a 5 cm incision is made upward along the midline from the pubic symphysis. The abdominal muscles are cut open along the linea alba abdominis and the bladder is moved outside. A "purse string suture" is performed by passing a thread through the bladder muscles in a circle pattern around a spot where there are fewer blood vessels, and then a small incision in the centre of this circle is made. The bladder cannula is inserted through the cut into the bladder, then the purse string suture is tightened around the end of the bladder cannula. After the cannula is inserted, its end is placed on a petri dish. The incision should be covered with warm gauze soaked by normal saline after operation (Fig. 3 – 12).

(2) Duodenum cannulation   The hair on the middle of the upper abdomen is sheared. A 6 – 7 cm incision is made downward along the midline from the sternum xiphoid process. After the abdominal cavity is opened, the duodenum is found, under which the silk threads are passed. Then a small opening is cut in the intestinal wall and a canula is inserted about 4 cm into the duodenum, which is fixed with suture threads. The intestines are put back into the cavity and the abdominal wall is closed with forceps.

(Zhang Na   Daniel H. Nissen)

第四章　基础及综合性实验

实验一　刺激强度和刺激频率与骨骼肌收缩反应的关系

【实验目的】　掌握蟾蜍（或蛙）坐骨神经-腓肠肌标本的制备方法；观察不同刺激强度和刺激频率对骨骼肌收缩的影响。

【实验原理】　给予骨骼肌施加一次足够强的单刺激时，可引起骨骼肌产生一次单收缩。单收缩是机体所有正常收缩的基础，因此对单收缩的研究也是非常重要的。骨骼肌收缩产生的张力决定于同时发生反应的运动单位（一个脊髓前角运动神经元及其轴突分支所支配的全部肌纤维，称为一个运动单位）数量的多少。增大刺激强度可以增加同时产生收缩的运动单位的数量，当刺激强度增大到一定数值时，所有的运动单位都兴奋，肌张力也达到最大，再增大刺激强度，肌张力不会随刺激强度的增大而增大，这一过程称为运动单位的总和。

当给骨骼肌施加一连串的刺激时，刺激的时间间隔大于一个单收缩的收缩期和舒张期之和时，可产生一连串的相互分开的单收缩。刺激频率增加时，刺激间隔缩短，如果间隔时间大于收缩期而小于收缩期和舒张期之和时，后一刺激引起的肌肉收缩落在前一刺激引起的收缩过程的舒张期内，出现不完全强直收缩。进一步增大刺激频率，后一刺激引起的收缩将落在前一刺激引起肌肉收缩的缩短期内，没有舒张期的出现，形成完全强直收缩。对不同的标本而言，产生强直收缩所需的刺激频率可能不同。

【实验对象】　蟾蜍

【实验用品】　BL－420生物机能实验系统，张力换能器，蛙类常用手术器械，林格液

【实验步骤】

1. 坐骨神经-腓肠肌标本的制备

（1）破坏脑和脊髓　左手握住蟾蜍，用示指按压头部前端，拇指按压背部，使头前俯；右手持金属探针由头前端沿中线向尾方刺触，触及凹陷处即枕骨大孔。将探针由凹陷处垂直刺入枕骨大孔并将尖端转向头端刺入颅腔，横向搅动捣毁脑组织；然后退出探针至皮下转向尾方，与脊柱平行刺入椎管破坏脊髓。如蛙四肢松弛，呼吸停止，表示破坏完全，如图4－1所示。

（2）剪除躯干上部及内脏　在蛙骶髂关节水平以上1 cm处，用粗剪刀剪断脊柱，并将头和前肢连同内脏剪去。在腹侧脊柱两侧可见到坐骨神经，如图4－2所示。

（3）剥皮　用镊子夹住脊柱断端（不要夹住或接触神经），右手捏紧皮肤边缘，向下撕掉后肢的全部皮肤，然后将标本放入盛有林格液的培养皿中，如图4－3所示。将手和用过的器械洗净擦干。

（4）游离坐骨神经　将标本背位固定于蛙板上，循股二头肌和半膜肌之间的坐骨神经沟，用玻璃分针纵向分离出坐骨神经股骨段直至腘窝。在坐骨神经由脊柱发出的部位用丝线结扎，并在近脊柱侧用眼科剪剪断神经。轻提结扎线，剪断坐骨神经的所有小分支，游离至腘窝。

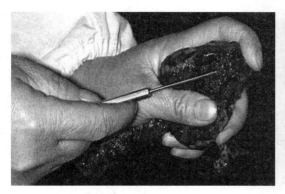

图 4 - 1　破坏蛙的脑和脊髓

Fig. 4 - 1　Destroy the brain and spinal cord

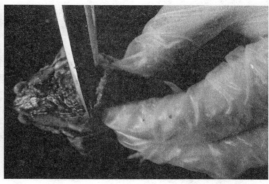

图 4 - 2　剪除蛙的躯干上部和内脏

Fig. 4 - 2　Cut away the upper body and internal organs

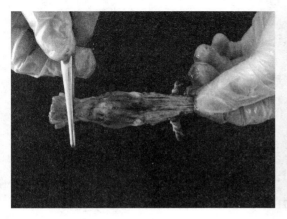

图 4 - 3　剥皮

Fig. 4 - 3　Skin peeling

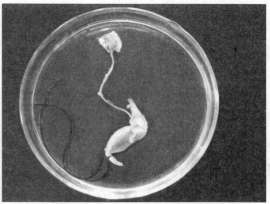

图 4 - 4　坐骨神经-腓肠肌标本

Fig. 4 - 4　Sciatic nerve-gastrocnemius muscle sample

（5）完成坐骨神经-腓肠肌标本　将分离干净的坐骨神经置于腓肠肌上，在膝关节周围剪断全部大腿肌肉，用粗剪刀将股骨刮干净，在股骨上中 1/3 处剪断（保留下 2/3 股骨）。在跟腱处用丝线结扎，在其远端剪断并游离腓肠肌至膝关节处，在膝关节以下将小腿其余部分全部剪除，得到坐骨神经-腓肠肌标本，如图 4 - 4 所示。将制备的坐骨神经-腓肠肌标本置于林格液中 5～10 min，待其兴奋性稳定后进行实验。

2. 仪器连接

（1）将张力换能器和肌动器分别用双凹夹固定在滴定架上、下方，并将前者接至 BL - 420 生物机能实验系统的相应通道。将刺激输出线与肌动器接线柱相连。

（2）将标本的股骨干固定在肌动器上，坐骨神经置于肌动器的电极上，腓肠肌与张力换能器应变片相连，调节双凹夹的位置使张力适度。

（3）单击"输入信号"菜单──→选定相应"通道"──→选择"张力"──→单击"开始"，开始实验

【观察项目】

1. 刺激强度与骨骼肌收缩力间的关系

（1）阈刺激　选单刺激，刺激强度从零开始，逐渐增大刺激强度，记录肌肉收缩曲线，

刚刚出现肌肉收缩波时的刺激为阈刺激。

（2）阈上刺激　选单刺激，在阈刺激基础上逐渐增大刺激强度记录收缩曲线，观察刺激强度与肌肉收缩力之间的关系。

（3）最大刺激　继续增大刺激强度，当肌肉收缩曲线不再随刺激强度增大而增高时的最小刺激强度即是最大刺激。

2. 刺激频率与骨骼肌收缩形式间的关系

（1）单收缩　选定并固定一个适宜的刺激强度（阈上刺激），给肌肉单刺激，观察记录收缩曲线。

（2）强直收缩　给神经肌肉标本连续刺激，逐渐增加刺激频率，观察不完全强直收缩和完全强直收缩并记录收缩曲线。

【注意事项】

1. 标本制备过程中，应尽量减少对神经和肌肉的损伤。

2. 对肌肉施加刺激时，刺激时间不要太长，一般不超过 4～6 s。

3. 在实验过程中要随时滴加林格液，防止标本干燥，保持其兴奋性。

【思考题】

1. 完全强直收缩和不完全强直收缩的产生机制是什么？

2. 标本制备过程中应注意什么？

（王小君　王银环）

Experiment 1　Effect of stimulation with different intensities and frequencies on muscular contraction

[**Experimental objectives**]　To grasp the method of sciatic‐gastrocnemius sample preparation; to observe the effect of stimulation with different intensities and frequencies on muscular contraction.

[**Experimental principles**]　A strong enough single stimulus to a skeletal muscle evokes a twitch, or a single contraction. As all of the normal body contractions are based on isolated single contractions, it is of significance to carry out the research on twitch contractions. The force generated by the muscular contractions depends on the number of motor units (a neuron and its muscle cells) that react simultaneously. Increasing the voltage used to stimulate the muscle will increase the number of motor units with simultaneous contractions. When stimulus intensity reaches to a particular level, then all motor units are excited and we will then get the maximum force producible. Afterwards, if the stimulus intensity is further increased, the muscle tension does not vary with the increased stimulus intensity. This is referred to as summation of motor units.

When the skeletal muscles receive a series of stimuli and the time interval between stimuli is greater than the sum of the contraction phase and the relaxation period of a single twitch, the twitches produced will be a series of separated individual contractions. When stimulation frequency increases, there will be a shortening of the time interval between stimuli. If the time interval between stimuli is greater than the contraction phase but shorter than the sum of the contraction phase and the relaxation period, then the muscle contraction induced by the following stimulus will occur during the relaxation period of the prior contraction process. This is referred to as incomplete tetanus. If the muscle is stimulated rapidly enough, succeeding contractions may come so close together that no relaxation occurs between contractions. When this occurs, the smooth state of contraction known as complete tetanus has been achieved. The frequency of stimulus necessary for complete tetanus varies depending on the particular muscle.

[**Experimental object**] toad

[**Experimental materials**] BL – 420 system, surgical instruments for toad, tension transducers, Ringer's solution

[**Experimental procedures**]

1. Preparation of sciatic nerve – gastrocnemius muscle sample

(1) Destroy the brain and spinal cord   Hold a toad with the left hand, press the front of its head and back with the thumb and forefinger. Hold the probe with the right hand and move the probe down alone the midline until the end of the skull. Prick the skin vertically at the hole of occipital bone, and then insert the of probe into the brain and destroy it. Then withdraw the probe to a point where the tip will be roughly positioned at the spinal cord and then swivel the tip around and insert into the canalis spinalis to destroy the spinal cord. The brain and spiral cord has been destroyed when the movement of the toad's four limbs and respiration disappears (Fig. 4 – 1).

(2) Cut away the upper body and internal organs   Use scissors to cut the toad's spine at a position 1 cm higher than the horizontal line of articulationes sacroiliac. Discard the head, forelimbs and viscus and only keep the small section of the back spine, hind legs and the sciatic nerve in both sides of spine (Fig. 4 – 2).

(3) Peel off the skin of the toad   Hold the broken parts of the spinal cord with the left hand and pinch the skin of the hind legs and peel off the skin. Put the sample into the glass with Ringer's solution. Then clean your hands and the used instruments (Fig. 4 – 3).

(4) Free the sciatic nerve   Fix the sample on the frog board with pins. Separate the sciatic nerve along the spiral cord, tie the end of it and cut it away. Lift the ligation thread lightly and cut the branch of the nerve. Separate the sciatic nerve from the sciatic nerve ditch with a glass dissecting needle, hold the thread, cut off all the branches to the knee joint.

(5) Finish the sciatic nerve – gastrocnemius muscle sample   Put the sciatic nerve on the fibula muscle and cut off all the thigh muscles around the knee joint. Scrape the thighbone with big scissors and shear off the thighbone (retain 2/3 of the lower part). Ligate the muscle at Achille's tendon, cut away the fibula muscle and separate it, and cut away the other part below the knee joint. Now the preparation of the sample is completed (Fig. 4 – 4). Immerse the sample into Ringer's solution for about 10 min.

2. Sample fixation and equipment connection

(1) Fix the thighbone sample in a hole near the electrode, put the fibula muscle above

the thighbone, connect the ligation thread with a hook on the head of transducer, and put the sciatic nerve on the electrode. The tension transducer is connected to the corresponding channel of BL - 420 system.

(2) Connect the electronic stimulator with electrode.

(3) Start BL - 420 software: click "input signal" menu and select "tension" in the submenu of the corresponding "channel".

[**Observations**]

1. Correlations between stimulus intensity and the force of skeletal muscles contractions

Give the specimen a weak stimulus (single pulse mode) and increase the stimulation intensity gradually till you are able to record the twitch curve—this intensity is the threshold intensity. Initially, if you keep on increasing the intensity, the twitch scale continues to increase. When the stimulation intensity reaches a certain level, the twitch scale will no longer increase with the stimulation intensity. This stimulation intensity is the most suitable intensity and this stimulus is the max stimulus.

2. Correlations between frequency of stimulation and the pattern of skeletal muscle contractions

The muscle is stimulated with an up-threshold stimulus first once per second (sequential pulse mode); the sample is allowed to rest for 15s and then the process is repeated instead with a stimulus firing rate of twice per second. If you gradually increase the frequency and stimulate the muscle, you will obtain summation, or an increased shortening of the muscle due to "overlap" of contractions. Normally, tetanus will occur with about 20~35 stimulations per second.

[**Precautions**]

1. Master the method of sciatic nerve-muscle. Do not destroy the samples. Do not touch the sample with your hands when separating the sample; instead, the sample should only be touched with glass rods. Do not pull the nerve excessively when separating.

2. Do not stimulate the sample too long, generally not more than 4 - 6 s.

3. Moisten the sample with Ringer solution, in order to keep it functioning well.

[**Questions**]

1. What is the mechanism of incomplete tetanus and complete tetanus?

2. What should be paid attention to in the process of specimen preparation?

(Wang Xiaojun)

实验二　蛙心起搏点的观察

【实验目的】　用结扎法观察两栖类动物心脏的起搏点和心脏不同部位传导系统的自动节律性高低。

【实验原理】　心脏特殊传导系统的各部分具有自律性，但自律性高低不同。两栖类动物的心脏起搏点是静脉窦（哺乳动物的起搏点是窦房结）。正常情况下，静脉窦（窦房结）的自律性最高，产生的节律性兴奋可依次传到心房、房室交界区、心室，引起整个心脏兴奋和收缩，因此静脉窦（窦房结）被称为正常起搏点；其他部位的自律组织仅起着兴奋传导作用，故称之为潜在起搏点。当静脉窦（窦房结）的兴奋传导受阻时，心房或心室受当时自律性最高部位发出的兴奋节律支配而搏动。

【实验对象】　蛙或蟾蜍

【实验用品】　蛙类常用手术器械一套，蛙板，图钉，玻璃分针，滴管，林格液

【实验步骤】

1. 破坏脑和脊髓　用探针破坏蛙的脑和脊髓后，仰卧固定在蛙板上。

2. 暴露心脏　剪开剑突处皮肤，用镊子夹住剑突，在剑突下剪一"V"形口并延续剪开胸腔，去掉胸骨，剪开心包膜，暴露心脏。

3. 识别蛙心结构　心脏腹面识别静脉窦、心房、心室，如图 4-5 所示。用玻璃分针将心尖翻向头端，从背面辨认，见心房与静脉窦之间有半月形白线为窦房沟。在主动脉干下穿线（斯氏第一结扎）备用，如图 4-6 所示。

【观察项目】

1. 观察静脉窦、心房、心室收缩的顺序，记录它们的搏动频率。

2. 结扎心脏背面窦房沟处预先穿入的线（即斯氏第一结扎），观察静脉窦、心房、心室的搏动频率。

3. 待心房、心室复跳后，再分别记录心房、心室的搏动频率。

4. 在心房与心室之间即房室沟做第二结扎（即斯氏第二结扎），记录静脉窦、心房、心室的搏动频率。将所有记录结果填入表 4-1。

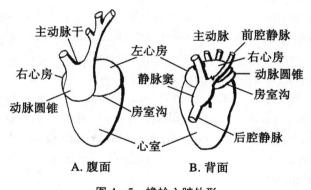

A. 腹面　　　B. 背面

图 4-5　蟾蜍心脏外形

Fig. 4-5　Shape of the toad heart

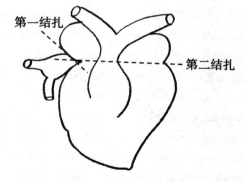

图 4-6　斯氏结扎部位

Fig. 4-6　Deligation sites

表 4-1　心脏各部分活动频率

Tab. 4 - 1   Frequency of venous sinus, atrium and ventricle (beats/min)

实验条件 Condition	静脉窦（次/min） Venous sinus	心房（次/min） Atrium	心室（次/min） Ventricle
结扎前状态 Before deligation			
斯氏第一结扎 First deligation			
斯氏第二结扎 Second deligation			

【注意事项】

1. 结扎前要认真识别心脏的结构。

2. 结扎部位要准确，结扎应迅速扎紧，使心房或心室搏动停止。

3. 实验中滴加林格液，保持心脏湿润。

【思考题】

1. 为什么正常起搏点能主导心脏的节律性活动？

2. 第一结扎后和第二结扎后心室搏动频率是否相同？为什么？

（张一兵　Daniel H. Nissen）

Experiment 2　Observation of cardiac pacemaker in toads

〔**Experimental objectives**〕　To observe the heart pacemaker in toads and identify the differences in auto-rhythmicity for different parts of the heart by means of deligation.

〔**Experimental principles**〕　The conducting system of the heart contains specialized auto - rhythmic cells, with different levels of rhythmicity in different parts of the heart. The venous sinus is the heart pacemaker in toads (sinus node for mammals). In the normal state, venous sinus can produce auto - rhythmic excitation which is the highest level of autorhythmicity in the heart. The excitation is transmitted to atrium, atrioventricular junction and ventricle in order to cause the heart excitation and contraction. Venous sinus is called the normal pacemaker to control the whole heart excitation and pulsation, and other rhythmic tissues are known as latent pacemakers since they usually only conduct the excitation and do not act as pacemakers except when the input stimulation is interrupted or the frequency is lower than its own self autorhythmicity frequency.

〔**Experimental object**〕　toad

〔**Experimental materials**〕　frog board, surgical instruments for toad, nail, glass dissecting needle, dropper, Ringer's solution

〔**Experimental procedures**〕

1. Destroy the brain and spinal cord　Destroy the brain and spinal cord of a toad and fix it on frog board in the supine position.

2. Expose the heart　Carry out the skin incision on the xiphisternum and make a V-shaped cut under the xiphisternum. Remove the sternum and open the cardiac pericardium

to expose the heart.

3. Identify the toad's heart structure   Identify the venous sinus, atrium and ventricle from ventral aspect of heart (Fig. 4 – 5), and then turn up the heart by glass needle to recognize the crescent-shaped groove (sino-atrial groove) between atrium and venous sinus. A suture is put under truncus aortae for future use (Fig. 4 – 6).

[**Observational items**]

1. Observe the systole order of venous sinus, atrium and ventricle and record their beating frequency.

2. Conduct the first deligation by using suture across sino-atrial groove. Observe the different beating frequencies of the venous sinus, atrium and ventricle frequency respectively.

3. When heartbeat resumes in atrium and ventricle, observe the atrium and ventricle beating frequencies respectively.

4. Conduct the second deligation by using suture across the atrioventricular groove. Observe the different beating frequencies of sinus venous, atrium and ventricle frequency respectively.   Fill all the results in Tab. 4 – 1.

[**Precautions**]

1. The heart structure must be recognized carefully before deligation.

2. Deligation must be fastened quickly in the correct site to stop heartbeat.

3. Ringer's solution should be dripped continuously to keep the heart moist.

[**Questions**]

1. Why does the normal peacemaker dominate the heart rhythmicity?

2. Is the frequency of the ventricle after the first deligation the same as that after the second deligation? Why?

(Zhang Yibing)

实验三　期前收缩和代偿间歇

【实验目的】　学习在体蛙心收缩活动曲线的记录方法；通过期前收缩和代偿间歇的观察，验证心肌有效不应期特别长的特征，从而加深对心肌兴奋性周期性变化特点的理解。

【实验原理】　心肌每发生一次兴奋后，其兴奋性会发生一系列周期性的变化。与其他可兴奋组织相比，心肌的有效不应期特别长，一直延续到心肌舒张活动的早期。在此期间，无论给予心肌多么强大的刺激，它也不会发生兴奋和收缩。因此，心肌不会像骨骼肌那样发生完全强直收缩。如果在心室肌的有效不应期后、下一次窦房结兴奋到达前，心室受到一次阈上刺激，则可提前产生一次兴奋和收缩，分别称为期前兴奋和期前收缩。期前兴奋也有其自身的有效不应期，当紧接在期前兴奋后的一次窦房结兴奋传到心室时，如果正好落在期前兴奋的有效不应期内，则此次正常下传的窦房结兴奋将不能引起心室的兴奋和收缩，即形成一次兴奋和收缩的"脱失"，须待下一次窦房结的兴奋传来时才能引起心室兴奋和收缩。这样，在一次期前收缩之后往往会出现一段较长的心室舒张期，称为代偿间歇。

【实验对象】　蟾蜍或蛙

【实验用品】 BL－420 生物机能实验系统，张力换能器，刺激电极，铁支架，双凹夹，蛙类手术器械，探针，蛙板，图钉，蛙心夹，缝合线，小烧杯，滴管，林格液

【实验步骤】

1. 破坏脑和脊髓　用探针破坏蛙或蟾蜍的脑和脊髓，将其仰卧固定于蛙板上。

2. 暴露心脏　从剑突下向上"V"形剪开皮肤，然后沿切口剪开胸骨、肋骨，打开胸腔，剪开心包暴露心脏。

3. 连接装置　将与张力换能器相连的蛙心夹在心室舒张期夹住心尖约 1 mm，调节双凹夹的位置使之有适当的张力，两个刺激电极分别夹在与蛙心夹相连的铜丝上和心脏周围的肌肉上。打开计算机，进入 BL－420 生物机能实验系统，点击"菜单"栏中输入信号，选择"通道"，"张力"信号，单击"开始"。

【观察项目】

1. 描记心脏正常收缩曲线，辨认曲线中代表收缩期和舒张期的部分。

2. 在心室收缩期，给予 3～5 V 的单次电刺激，观察心脏收缩曲线有无变化。

3. 在心室舒张早、中、晚期，分别给予 3～5 V 的单次电刺激，观察心脏收缩曲线有何变化？是否出现期前收缩和代偿间歇？

【注意事项】

1. 破坏蛙或蟾蜍的脑和脊髓要彻底。

2. 经常滴加林格液于心脏表面，以防止心脏组织干燥。

3. 不要连续刺激心脏。

【思考题】

1. 期前收缩后一定会出现代偿间歇吗？为什么？

2. 心肌的有效不应期特别长有何生理意义和临床意义？

（段国贤）

Experiment 3　Premature contraction and compensatory pause

[**Experimental objectives**]　To learn how to record the curve of toad heartbeat in vivo; to confirm the characteristics of cardiac muscle's long effective refractory period through observing premature contraction and compensatory pause; to obtain a further knowledge of the periodic changes of cardiac muscle's excitability.

[**Experimental principles**]　Once cardiac muscle excites, its excitability will change periodically. The effective refractory period of cardiac muscle is comparatively long, which almost equals to the whole length of systole and pre-diastole. During this period, any stronger stimulus can not cause the cardiac muscle to excite and contract. Therefore, the cardiac muscle have no tetanic contraction as skeletal muscles do. If the ventricle is given a suprathreshold stimulus after effective refractory period and before the next normal impulse from the sinoatrial node, it will excite and contract before the normal rhythmicity excitation. This is called premature excitation and contraction. Premature contraction also has the effective refractory period. If the normal rhythmic excitation conducting to ventricle from the sinoatrial node (venous sinus in toad) is exactly right in the effective refractory period of premature excitation, it cannot lead to ventricle's excitation and contraction, and the ventricle is in diastole. It is not until the next normal rhythmic excitation arrives that the ventricle recovers to normal rhythmic contraction. This long period of diastole after the premature systole is called compensatory pause.

[**Experimental object**] toad

[**Experimental materials**] BL – 420 experimental system, tension transducer, stimulation electrode, iron bracket, biconcave clamp, surgical instruments for toad, probe, frog board, nail, toad heart clip, suture, little beaker, dropper, Ringer's solution.

[**Experimental procedures**]

1. Destroy the brain and spinal cord Destroy the toad's brain and spinal cord by a probe, and put the toad on its back on the frog board.

2. Expose the heart Cut the skin from xiphisternum and make an inverted triangular incision. Open the thoracic cavity and cut the pericardium to expose the heart.

3. Connect the instruments Clip the apex of the heart for 1 mm in the diastole with a toad heart clip connected with a tension transducer. Adjust the site of the biconcave clamp for a moderate tension. Fix one of stimulus electrodes to brass wire connected with heart clip, the other one to the muscles around the heart. Turn on the computer and BL – 420 biology experimental system, click "input signal" to select the channel and "tension" signal. Click "start" button to start experiment.

[**Observations**]

1. Record a period of normal cardiac curves and recognize the curve of systole and diastole.

2. Give a single stimulus of 3 – 5 V during ventricle systole to observe the contraction of the ventricle.

3. During the early, intermediate and late period of diastole, give a single stimulus of 3 – 5 V respectively to see if the premature contraction and compensatory pause occur.

[**Precautions**]

1. Thoroughly destroy the brain and spinal cord.

2. Drip the Ringer's solution to keep the heart moist during the experiment.

3. Don't stimulate the heart constantly.

[**Questions**]

1. Does the compensatory pause always appear after premature contraction? Why?

2. What is the physiological and clinical significance of the long effective refractory period of cardiac muscles?

(Duan Guoxian)

实验四　红细胞渗透脆性

【实验目的】　通过观察红细胞在不同浓度低渗盐溶液中发生的变化，加深理解细胞外液渗透压的相对恒定对维持细胞正常形态与生理功能的重要性。

【实验原理】　0.9%的 NaCl 溶液与血浆等渗。将红细胞置于 0.9% 的 NaCl 溶液中，其形态和大小保持不变。若将红细胞置于低渗的 NaCl 溶液中，水将在渗透压的作用下进入细胞而使其膨胀甚至破裂，这一特性称为红细胞的渗透脆性。正常红细胞对低渗溶液有一定的抵抗能力，临床上常用不同浓度的 NaCl 溶液来检测红细胞的渗透脆性。当 NaCl 浓度降至 0.42% 时，部分红细胞开始破裂而发生溶血，此 NaCl 浓度为红细胞的最小渗透抵抗力。当 NaCl 浓度降至 0.35% 时，则全部红细胞发生溶血，该 NaCl 浓度为红细胞的最大渗透抵抗力。对低渗溶液的抵抗力越小，表示红细胞的渗透脆性越大；相反，对低渗溶液的抵抗力越大，表示红细胞的渗透脆性越小。生理情况下，初成熟的红细胞的渗透脆性小而衰老的红细胞大一些。遗传性球形红细胞增多症和镰状红细胞增多症患者的红细胞脆性增大。

【实验对象】　家兔

【实验用品】　试管架，10 ml 试管 9 支，2 ml 注射器 1 支，滴管，5 ml 吸管 2 支，3.8% 枸橼酸钠，1% NaCl 溶液，蒸馏水

【实验步骤】

1. 制备不同浓度的 NaCl 溶液　取试管 9 支，编号，依次排列在试管架上，按表 4 - 2 配制不同浓度的 NaCl 溶液，混匀。

2. 兔血的制备　麻醉状态下行家兔颈总动脉插管，取兔血 2 ml，加入装有 3.8% 枸橼酸钠溶液 0.2 ml 的试管中，混匀备用。

3. 红细胞悬液的制备　用滴管向每支试管中滴加兔血 2 滴，轻轻摇匀，静置 1 h 后观察每个试管中颜色、透明度有何差别。

表 4 - 2　不同浓度 NaCl 溶液的配制

Tab. 4 - 2　The preparation of NaCl solutions of different concentrations

试管编号 Number	1	2	3	4	5	6	7	8	9
1% NaCl（ml）Volume of NaCl solution	3.6	2.6	2.2	2.0	1.8	1.6	1.4	1.2	—
蒸馏水（ml）Volume of distilled water	0.4	1.4	1.8	2.0	2.2	2.4	2.6	2.8	4.0
NaCl 浓度（%）Concentration of NaCl solution	0.90	0.60	0.55	0.50	0.45	0.40	0.35	0.3	—

【观察项目】

请按下列标准进行观察：

1. 试管内液体分层，上层为无色或淡黄色透明液体，下层为浑浊红色，表示没有溶血。

2. 试管内液体分层，上层呈红色透明液体，下层为浑浊红色，表示部分红细胞破裂溶解，为不完全溶血。最先出现不完全溶血的试管中溶液的浓度代表红细胞的最小渗透抵抗力。

3. 管内液体完全变成透明的红色，管底无细胞沉积，表明红细胞全部破裂，为完全溶血，最先出现完全溶血的试管中溶液的浓度代表红细胞的最大渗透抵抗力。

【注意事项】

1. 试管一定要编号，以免混淆。

2. 向试管中加入血液时，要靠近液面，使血液轻轻滴入溶液中，滴入血液后轻轻摇匀，避免剧烈震荡，以免溶血。

3. 吸不同溶液的吸管，必须严格区分，不得混用。

4. 取液量要准确，以确保试管中溶液的浓度精确。

【思考题】

1. 临床大量输液时为何要输等张溶液？

2. 哪些因素可影响红细胞的渗透脆性？为什么同一家兔的不同红细胞对低渗溶液的抵抗力大小不同？

3. 哪些因素可影响红细胞渗透脆性实验的准确性？

（段国贤）

Experiment 4　Osmotic fragility of erythrocytes

〔**Experimental objectives**〕　To learn the significance of relative constant osmotic pressure of extracellular fluid in keeping the normal shape and functions of cells by observing the erythrocyte changes in different osmotic solutions.

〔**Experimental principles**〕　The osmotic pressure of 0.9％ NaCl solution is equal to that of plasma. The shape and volume of erythrocytes remain the same when suspended in isotonic NaCl solution. However, if the erythrocytes are suspended in a hypotonic solution, the water will permeate into the cells to make them bulge and break. This characteristic is called osmotic fragility. Normal erythrocytes have resistance to hypotonic solutions. Hypotonic NaCl solutions of different concentrations are generally used to test the erythrocyte fragility in clinic. Normal erythrocytes have a minimum osmotic resistance of 0.42％ NaCl solution in which some of the erythrocytes begin to dissolve and maximum osmotic resistance of 0.35％ NaCl solution in which they all break. The smaller the erythrocytes resistances to the hypotonic solutions are, the bigger their osmotic fragility will be. On the contrary, the bigger the erythrocytes resistances to the hypotonic solution are, the smaller their osmotic fragility will be. Physiologically, the osmotic fragility of young erythrocytes is relatively small while that of old erythrocytes is much larger. The osmotic fragility of erythrocytes will increase in the patients with genetic spherocytic erythromatosis or drepanocytic polycythemia.

〔**Experimental object**〕　rabbit

〔**Experimental materials**〕　tubes rack, 9 test tubes (10 ml), 1 syringe (2 ml), 1 dropper, 2 pipettes (5 ml), sodium citrate solution (3.8％), 1％ NaCl solution, distilled water

〔**Experimental procedures**〕

1. Prepare NaCl solutions of different concentrations　Take 9 test tubes and assemble them on the rack after numbering them. Prepare NaCl solutions of different concentrations as Tab. 4 - 2. Mix up the solutions.

2. Prepare rabbit blood　Carotid artery cannulation is performed under anesthesia. Take 2 ml rabbit blood and mix it up with 0. 2 ml sodium citrate solution （3. 8%） in a test tube.

3. Prepare erythrocyte suspension　Add 2 drops of blood into each test tube and gently shake the tubes respectively. Allow the tubes to sit for an hour, and then observe the differences in color and transparency for each tube.

[Observations]

Observe the tubes and decide which one of the following applies：

1. Liquid layer in vitro. If the upper clear liquid is achromatic color and the bottom in the tube is turbid with red color, there is no hemolysis.

2. Liquid layer in vitro. If the upper clear liquid is pale red and the bottom in the tube is turbid with red color, there is an incomplete hemolysis with some of the erythrocytes dissolved. The concentration of NaCl solution when hemolysis first appears is the minimum osmotic resistance of erythrocyte.

3. If the liquid in the tube is completely clear and red, and there are not any cells on the bottom, it is called complete hemolysis. The concentration of NaCl solution when complete hemolysis first appears is the maximum osmotic resistance of erythrocyte.

[Precautions]

1. Do number the tubes to avoid confusion.

2. Approach to the liquid surface as near as possible, the blood gently into the solution and shake the tube lightly to avoid hemolysis.

3. The pipettes used to take different solutions must be distinguished strictly without being mixed for use.

4. Ensure the exact concentration of the solution in each of the tubes by taking the accurately measuring the volume of liquids.

[Questions]

1. Why are the isotonic solutions needed in clinical transfusion?

2. What can influence the osmotic fragility of erythrocytes? Why different erythrocytes in the same rabbit have different resistance to the hypotonic solutions?

3. What can influence the accuracy of the test of osmotic fragility of erythrocytes?

(Duan Guoxian)

实验五　胸内负压和气胸的观察

【实验目的】　学习胸内负压的测定方法；观察不同因素对胸内负压的影响。

【实验原理】　胸内压指胸膜腔内的压力，通常低于大气压，称为胸内负压。胸膜腔内的压力在一个呼吸周期中是有变化的，平静呼吸时胸膜腔内的压力可随吸气和呼气而升降。在胸膜腔密闭性被破坏后，外界空气进入胸膜腔形成气胸，胸内负压就会消失。将穿刺针头用橡皮管与水检压计相连，刺入胸膜腔后，即可通过水检压计观察胸内压的变化。

【实验对象】　家兔

【实验用品】　兔手术台，哺乳动物手术器械一套，腰椎穿刺针，气管插管，水检压计和橡皮管，注射器和针头，25％氨基甲酸乙酯，生理盐水

【实验步骤】

1. 麻醉、固定　以25％氨基甲酸乙酯（4 ml/kg）经兔耳缘静脉注射，待其麻醉后仰卧位固定于兔手术台上。

2. 气管插管　剪去颈部和右侧胸部的毛。沿颈部正中线纵向切开皮肤，分离出气管，插入气管插管，用丝线固定。

3. 连接检压计　将腰椎穿刺针用橡皮管连接水检压计。在兔胸腋前线的第5肋骨上缘，将针头顺肋骨方向斜插入胸腔，如见水检压计的水柱面下降并随呼吸运动而上下波动，表明已经插入胸膜腔内。固定穿刺针，防止针头移位或滑出。

【观察项目】

1. 平静呼吸时的胸内压　记录平静呼吸运动2～3 min，待呼吸平稳后，从水检压计上读出胸内负压的数值，比较吸气和呼气时胸内负压数值的不同。

2. 增大无效腔对胸内负压的影响　将气管插管的一侧管接一短橡皮管，再予以夹闭；在另一侧管上接一长50 cm的橡皮管，以增大无效腔，使呼吸加深加快。观察并记录胸内压数值，此时胸内压与平静呼吸时有何不同。

3. 气道阻塞对胸内负压的影响　在吸气末和呼气末，分别堵塞气管插管侧管。此时动物用力呼吸，但不能吸入或呼出外界气体，处于憋气状态。观察并记录胸内压变动的最大幅度，呼气时胸内负压可否高于大气压。

4. 气胸对胸内负压的影响　于上腹部切开腹壁，将内脏下推，观察膈肌的运动，再沿第7肋骨上缘切开皮肤，分离肋间肌形成长约1 cm的创口，贯穿胸壁，使胸膜腔与外界大气相通，形成气胸。观察肺组织是否萎陷，胸内压是否仍低于大气压，此时的胸内压是否还随呼吸而升降。

5. 气胸的处理　形成气胸后，封闭贯穿胸壁的创口，并用注射器排出胸膜腔内的气体，观察胸内压的变化。

【注意事项】

1. 胸腔穿刺时不要插得过猛和过深，以防刺破肺组织和血管，形成气胸和血胸。

2. 穿刺过程中，针头刺入胸壁已相当深，但仍未见水柱面波动，要停止刺入。可将针头转动一下，或微微调整角度。如果仍无效，应拔出针头，检查是否有组织碎片或血凝块堵塞针头，疏通后再穿刺。

【思考题】

1. 平静呼吸时，胸内负压始终低于大气压，为什么？

2. 气胸时胸膜腔内压有何变化？为什么？

3. 在什么情况下胸膜腔内压高于大气压？为什么？

（王小君）

Experiment 5   Observation of intrapleural negative pressure and pneumothorax

[**Experimental objectives**]   To study the method of recording the negative pressure of intrapleural space; to observe the changes of intrapleural pressure during the course of respiration movement and pneumothorax.

[**Experimental principles**]   The pressure inside pleural cavity is called intrapleural negative pressure, which is usually lower than atmospheric pressure. Its numeric value changes during respiratory cycle. During eupnea the intrapleural negative pressure can increase and decrease between inspiration and expiration. When the chest wall is pierced, atmospheric air rushes into the intrapleural space, and the intrapleural negative pressure will disappear. If we connect the lumbar puncture needle with the water-pressure manometer using a rubber tube and insert the needle into pleural cavity, then we can observe the changes to the intrapleural negative pressure.

[**Experimental object**]   rabbit

[**Experimental materials**]   surgical instruments for mammalian, operating table for rabbit, tracheal cannula, syringe, rubber tube, lumbar puncture needle, water-pressure manometer, 25% urethan, normal saline

[**Experimental procedures**]

1. Anesthesia and rabbit restraint   Inject 25% urethane (4 ml/kg) into the marginal ear vein of the rabbit and fix it on the operating table in the supine body position after the rabbit has been anesthetized.

2. Tracheal cannulation   Shear the hair on the neck and the right chest. Cut the skin along the middle cervical line and separate the trachea from the surrounding tissues. Cut open the trachea and insert the tracheal cannula, and fix the tracheal cannula with threads.

3. Connect ion to the pressure manometer   Connect a lumbar puncture needle with water-pressure manometer. Insert the needle into the pleural cavity at the fifth costa in pectoral axillary front line. If the water column of water-pressure manometer decreases and fluctuates with respiration, it shows that the needle has been correctly inserted into the pleural cavity. Fix the needle on the skin with a sticking plaster.

[**Observations**]

1. Intrapleural pressure at eupnea   Record respiratory movements at eupnea for 2 - 3 minutes. When the respiration is steady, we can read the value of the intrapleural negative pressure from the water-pressure manometer. Measure intrapleural negative pressures and compare the difference of intrapleural negative pressure between inspiration and expiration.

2. The effect of increasing the dead space   On a branch of the tracheal cannula connect a short rubber tube and bend the tube back on to itself so as to block the air flow in that tube. On another branch of tracheal cannula connect a 50 cm rubber tube, and then the respi-

ration will be deepened and speeded up by enlarging the dead space. Observe and record the value of intrapleural negative pressures at deep breathing. Compare the difference of intrapleural pressure between deep breathing and eupnea.

3. The effect of airway obstruction　At end of inspiration and expiration，block the tracheal cannula for some seconds. Though the rabbit makes an effort to breathe，it cannot exhale or inhale air from the environment in this state of breathholding. Observe and record the maximum range of variation of intrapleural negative pressure. Observe whether intrapleural negative pressure is higher than atmospheric pressure during expiration.

4. The effect of pneumothorax　Cut the open abdominal wall from the upper abdomen and push the splanchna down，then observe the movement of the diaphragm muscle. Cut open skin along the superior border of the seventh rib and separate intercostal muscles with a hemostat to make a 1 cm wound running through the chest wall，through which air can go into the pleural cavity，and thus pneumothorax is formed. Observe whether lung collapse occurs；Whether intrapleural pressure is lower than atmosphere pressure and varies with respiration and what is the change of the intrapleural pressure.

5. Treatment of pneumothorax　When pneumothorax has been formed，block the wound quickly and draw out air from the pleural cavity with syringe. Observe whether the intrapleural pressure can recover from being positive.

[**Precautions**]

1. Do not insert the needle too fast or too deeply in case of cutting the lung and vessels with the result of pneumothorax or hemathorax.

2. Insertion should be stopped when the needle has penetrated deeply enough，even if the liquid level fluctuation is not observed. If it does not work，the needle should be pulled out and examined. If fragments of tissue or blood clot block the needle，clear it out and repeat the insertion.

[**Questions**]

1. Why is intrapleural pressure always lower than atmospheric pressure all the time at eupnea?

2. How will intrapleural pressure change when pneumothorax occurs? Why?

3. Under what conditions is the intrapleural pressure positive? Why?

(Wang Xiaojun)

实验六　呼吸运动的调节

【实验目的】　学习呼吸运动的记录方法；观察多种因素对家兔呼吸运动的影响。

【实验原理】　呼吸运动是呼吸中枢节律性活动的反应。在不同生理状况下，呼吸运动所做出的适应性变化有赖于各种神经反射的调节，其中比较重要的有通过中枢和外周化学感受器完成的反射以及肺牵张反射。体内外各种刺激可直接作用于呼吸中枢，或通过不同的感受器而反射性地影响呼吸运动。

【实验对象】 家兔

【实验用品】 BL－420 生物机能实验系统，哺乳动物手术器械，兔手术台，玛丽气鼓，张力换能器，气管插管，20 ml 和 5 ml 注射器各 1 个，50 cm 长乳胶管，纱布，手术线，CO_2 气囊，25％氨基甲酸乙酯，3％乳酸，生理盐水

【实验步骤】

1. 麻醉、固定　由耳缘静脉注射 25％氨基甲酸乙酯（4 ml/kg），待家兔麻醉后仰卧位固定于兔手术台上。

2. 手术　气管插管，分离双侧迷走神经。

3. 仪器连接及调试　将与张力换能器相连的玛丽气鼓的胶管与一侧气管插管连接。进入 BL－420 生物机能实验系统，点击"输入信号"，选择"通道"，点击"张力"信号，点击"开始"，开始实验。

【观察项目】

1. 正常的呼吸运动曲线

2. CO_2 对呼吸运动的影响　将气管插管的侧开口端与装有 CO_2 的气囊口相对，打开气囊皮管夹，使 CO_2 随吸气进入气管，观察增大吸入气中 CO_2 浓度对呼吸运动的影响。待呼吸运动出现明显变化时移去气囊使呼吸运动恢复正常。

3. 气道阻力对呼吸运动的影响　待家兔呼吸平稳后，部分阻塞一侧气管插管，观察气道阻力增大后呼吸运动的变化。

4. 无效腔对呼吸运动的影响　在气管插管侧口连接 50 cm 的乳胶管，观察无效腔增大后呼吸运动的变化。

5. 血液酸度对呼吸运动的影响　由耳缘静脉注入 3％乳酸 2 ml，观察呼吸运动的变化。

6. 迷走神经对呼吸运动的影响　先切断一侧迷走神经观察呼吸运动的改变，再切断另外一侧迷走神经，观察呼吸运动的变化。

【注意事项】

1. 描记正常的呼吸运动曲线作为对照，等家兔从上一观察项目恢复后再开始下一个观察项目。

2. 分离神经时注意不要损伤神经。

3. 当呼吸运动出现明显变化后，应立即终止作用因素，以恢复正常呼吸。

【思考题】

1. 电刺激迷走神经，呼吸运动会有何改变？

2. 耳缘静脉注射乳酸引起呼吸运动变化的机制是什么？

（张　伟）

Experiment 6　Regulation of respiratory movements in rabbits

[**Experimental objectives**]　To learn how to record respiratory movement; to observe the influences of various stimulus on respiratory movements in the rabbit.

[**Experimental principles**]　Respiratory movements are the reaction of rhythmical movement of respiratory center. In different physiological conditions, adaptive changes occuring in respiratory movements are dependent on the reflex adjustment of nervous system, in which the reflex adjustments of central and peripheral chemoreceptor and the pulmonary stretch reflex are more important than others. So no matter whether the stimulus factor origins from internal or external, it can change respiratory movements directly by affecting the respiration center or respiratory reflex .

[**Experimental object**]　rabbit

[**Experimental materials**]　BL – 420 experiment system, surgical apparatus, rabbit operating table, Mary's tambour, tension transducer, tracheal cannula, 20 ml and 5 ml syringes, rubber tube (50 cm), gauze, thread, carbon dioxide ballonet, 25% urethane, 3% lactic acid, 0. 9% NaCl solution

[**Experimental procedures**]

1. Anesthesia and fixation　25% urethane (4 ml/kg) is injected into the marginal ear vein of the rabbit's ear. And then fix the rabbit on the operation table in the supine body position after it has been anesthetized.

2. Operation　Insert the Y tracheal cannula and detach the bilateral vagus .

3. Instrument connection and configuration　Connect the branch of the tracheal cannula with the rubber tube connected to the mary' tambour which is linked to the tension transducer. Open BL – 420 system, click "input signal" to select the "channel" and "tension" signal. Click "start" button to start experiment.

[**Observations**]

1. The normal curve of respiratory movements.

2. Effect of CO_2 on respiratory movements　The peristome of the CO_2 ballonet was aimed to another opening of the tracheal cannula, then open screw clip on the ballonet to allow some CO_2 into trachea.

3. Effect of tracheal resistance on respiratory movements　When respiration is normal, partly block one side of the tracheal cannula and observe the change of respiration.

4. Effect of enlarging dead space on respiratory movements　Connect a 50 cm rubber tube with the other side of the tracheal cannula to enlarge the dead space, observe the change of respiration.

5. Effect of acid substance in blood on respiratory movements　Inject 3% Lactic acid 2 ml into the marginal ear vein of the rabbit and observe the change of respiration.

6. Effect of vagus nerve on respiratory movements　Cut off one side of vagus and then observe the change of respiration. Furthermore, cut off the other side of vagus and then observe the change of respiration.

[**Precautions**]

1. Record the normal curve as the control, and allow the rabbit to recover from the last experiment procedure before the next procedure.

2. Don't damage the nerves when separating them.

3. The affecting factors must be terminated immediately after significant changes occur in the respiration so as to recover to the normal breathing.

[Questions]

1. How will respiratory movements change when electrical stimulation is applied to the vagus?

2. What is the mechanism of respiratory change when lactic acid is injected into the rabbit by the ear vein?

（Zhang Wei）

实验七　胃肠道运动的观察

【实验目的】　观察正常情况下胃肠的运动形式以及神经体液因素对胃肠运动的影响。

【实验原理】　消化道平滑肌具有自动节律性，可以形成多种形式的运动，主要有紧张性收缩、蠕动、分节运动等。在整体内，消化道的运动受神经和体液的调节。副交感神经兴奋通过末梢释放乙酰胆碱加强胃肠运动，M受体阻断剂阿托品则抑制胃肠运动；交感神经兴奋时末梢释放去甲肾上腺素抑制胃肠运动。

【实验对象】　家兔

【实验用品】　哺乳类动物手术器械，兔手术台，保护电极，注射器，25％氨基甲酸乙酯，10^{-4} mol/L 肾上腺素溶液，10^{-4} mol/L 乙酰胆碱溶液，阿托品注射液，生理盐水。

【实验步骤】

1. 麻醉、固定　家兔称重，耳缘静脉注射 25％氨基甲酸乙酯（4 ml/kg）进行麻醉后，背位固定于兔手术台上。

2. 颈部手术　分离气管并做气管插管，分离一侧颈部迷走神经。

3. 腹部手术　沿腹部正中线，自剑突向下打开腹腔，暴露胃肠，以备观察。

【观察项目】

1. 观察正常情况下胃肠的运动。

2. 将迷走神经置于保护电极上，以 3～5 V，30～70 Hz 连续脉冲进行刺激，观察胃肠运动的变化。

3. 耳缘静脉注射 10^{-4} mol/L 肾上腺素溶液 0.5 ml，或直接滴加于胃和小肠的表面，观察胃肠运动的变化。

4. 耳缘静脉注射 10^{-4} mol/L 乙酰胆碱溶液 0.5 ml，或直接滴加于胃和小肠的表面，观察胃肠运动的变化。

5. 耳缘静脉注射阿托品 1 ml，或直接滴加于胃和小肠的表面，观察胃肠运动的变化。

【注意事项】

1. 操作轻柔，以免损伤胃肠或使其收缩。

2. 注意经常用温生理盐水溶液湿润胃肠表面，防止其干燥并保温。

【思考题】

1. 胃和小肠的运动形式有哪些？各有何生理意义？

2. 滴加乙酰胆碱与刺激迷走神经对胃肠运动影响的方式有何不同？

（孙　娜）

Experiment 7　Observation of gastrointestinal motility

[**Experimental objectives**]　To observe the forms of gastrointestinal motility under normal conditions and the influence of neural and humoral factors on it.

[**Experimental principles**]　Smooth muscles in the digestive tract have autorhythmicity and can produce many kinds of gastrointestinal motility, including tonic contraction, peristalsis and segmentation. In the body, gastrointestinal motility is regulated by the neural and humoral factors. Parasympathetic nerve can release acetylcholine which can stimulate gastrointestinal motility; Atropine, the blocker of M receptor, can inhibit gastrointestinal motility. Sympathetic nerve can reduce gastrointestinal motility by releasing norepinephrine.

[**Experimental object**]　rabbit

[**Experimental materials**]　surgical instruments for mammals, operation table for rabbit, shielded electrode, syringe, 25% urethane, 10^{-4} adrenalin solution, 10^{-4} acetylcholine solution, atropine solution, 0.9% normal saline.

[**Experimental procedures**]

1. Anesthesia and fixation　Catch a rabbit and weigh it, then anaesthetize the rabbit by injecting 25% urethane (4 ml/kg) through the marginal ear vein. Fix the rabbit on the operation table in the supine body position.

2. Operation on the neck　Separate the trachea and conduct the intubation, and separate the vagus nerve on one side of the neck.

3. Operation on the abdomen　Cut the skin below the ensisternum downwards along the midline and open the abdominal cavity. Then expose the stomach and intestines.

[**Observations**]

1. Observe the normal gastrointestinal motility.

2. Stimulate the vagus nerve by a shielded electrode, and observe the changes of gastrointestinal motility. The parameters of successive stimulus are as follows: intensity 3 – 5 V, frequency 30 – 70 Hz.

3. Inject 10^{-4} adrenalin 0.5 ml through the marginal ear vein or drip on the surface of stomach and intestines, and then observe the changes of gastrointestinal motility.

4. Inject 10^{-4} acetylcholine solution 0.5 ml through the marginal ear vein or drip on the surface of stomach and intestines, and then observe the changes of gastrointestinal motility.

5. Inject atropine solution 1ml through the marginal ear vein or drip on the surface of stomach and intestines, and then observe the changes of gastrointestinal motility.

[**Precautions**]

1. Operate gently and carefully, and avoid the injury or the contraction of the stomach and intestines.

2. Keep the surface of stomach and intestines warm and moist.

1. What's the motility mode of the stomach and intestines? What's the physiological significance?

2. What's the difference in terms of the influence on the gastrointestinal motility between the acetylcholine dripping on the surface and electrical stimulus on vagus nerve?

(Sun Na)

实验八　尿生成的影响因素

【实验目的】　学会用膀胱插管术收集尿液；以尿量为观察指标，观察各种因素对尿生成的影响，并分析其机制。

【实验原理】　尿的生成包括肾小球滤过、肾小管和集合管的重吸收、肾小管和集合管的分泌三个基本环节。凡影响上述过程的因素，均能影响尿的生成，从而引起尿量及尿液成分的改变。

【实验对象】　家兔

【实验用品】　哺乳类动物手术器械，兔手术台，膀胱插管，气管插管，头皮针，注射器，25％氨基甲酸乙酯，10^{-4} mol/L 去甲肾上腺素，呋塞米，20％葡萄糖溶液，垂体后叶素，0.6％酚红，10％ NaOH，尿糖试纸，生理盐水

【实验步骤】

1. 麻醉、固定　家兔称重，25％氨基甲酸乙酯（4 ml/kg）耳缘静脉注射麻醉，然后背位固定于兔手术台上。

2. 气管插管　在颈部正中分离气管并插管。

3. 膀胱插管　腹部正中剪毛，耻骨联合向上沿腹正中切开皮肤 5 cm。沿腹白线切开腹壁肌肉，将膀胱移至腹腔外。在膀胱顶部选择血管较少处做一荷包缝合进行膀胱插管。

【观察项目】

1. 记录麻醉状态下的尿量。

2. 先用尿糖试纸做尿糖定性试验，然后耳缘静脉注射 20％葡萄糖溶液 10 ml，观察尿量的变化。当尿量改变明显时，再做尿糖定性试验，并记录尿量。

3. 耳缘静脉注射 10^{-4} mol/L 去甲肾上腺素 0.3 ml，观察尿量的变化。

4. 耳缘静脉注射呋塞米 5 mg/kg，观察尿量的变化。

5. 耳缘静脉注射 0.6％的酚红 1 ml，用盛有 10％NaOH 的培养皿收集尿液，观察颜色的变化，如果尿液中有酚红排出，遇 NaOH 溶液即呈现玫瑰紫色。记录从开始注射酚红到尿中排出酚红所需要的时间，即酚红排泄时间。

6. 耳缘静脉注射垂体后叶素 2 U，观察尿量的变化。

【注意事项】

1. 实验前给予家兔足够量的水，以保证基础尿量。

2. 干预因素的实施要按照实验步骤顺序进行，不能颠倒。

3. 用注射器抽取药物，不能将药物混合。

4. 除麻醉外，其他静脉给药均采用留置头皮针进行。

【思考题】

1. 给家兔耳缘静脉注射生理盐水 20 ml，尿量有何变化？分析其原因。
2. 在影响尿生成的因素实验中，应注意哪些问题？

（李树民）

Experiment 8　Factors influencing the urine formation

〔**Experimental objectives**〕　To study bladder cannulation for collecting urine; to observe the factors influencing the urine formation and analyze the mechanisms of these factors.

〔**Experimental principles**〕　Formation of urine involves three basic processes: ultrafiltration of plasma by the glomerulus, selective reabsorption from the ultrafiltration and secretion of selected solutes into the tubular fluid by tubular and collecting duct. The factors that affect the above-mentioned processes of urine formation can change the volume and composition of urine.

〔**Experimental object**〕　rabbit

〔**Experimental materials**〕　surgical instruments for mammals, operation table for rabbit, bladder cannula, tracheal cannula, scalp venous needle, syringe, 25% urethane, 10^{-4} mol/L norepinephrine (NE), furosemide, 20% glucose solution, antidiuretic hormone (ADH), 0.6% phenol red (PR), 10% NaOH, Tes-Tape (test paper), 0.9% normal saline (NaCl)

〔**Experimental procedures**〕

1. Anesthesia and fixation　Weigh the rabbit and anesthetize it by administration of 25% urethane (4 ml/kg) through the marginal ear vein. And then fix it in the supine body position on the operating table.

2. Tracheal cannulation　Separate the trachea on the middle of the neck and perform intubation.

3. Bladder cannulation　Shear the hair on the inferior belly; make a 5 cm incision upward along middle line from the pubic symphysis. Cut abdominal wall along linea alba abdomin and move the bladder outside. Purse string suture is made in a place where there are fewer blood vessels to perform cannulation.

〔**Observations**〕

1. Record the normal urine volume.

2. Conduct the qualitative test for glucose in urine first before injecting glucose solution. Observe the result of normal urine. Administer 20% glucose solution 10 ml via the marginal ear vein. Observe the change of urine volume. When urine volume changes markedly, record the urine volume and conduct the qualitative test again.

3. Inject 10^{-4} mol/L norepinephrine 0.3 ml into the marginal ear vein. Observe the change of urine volume.

4. Inject furosemide 5 mg/kg into the marginal ear vein. Observe the change of urine volume.

5. Inject 0.6% phenol red 1 ml and allow the urine drip into a petri dish with some 10%

55

NaOH inside. Phenol red turns into rose-purple when it mixes with NaOH. Observe the change of color carefully, and record the time from the injection to the appearance of phenol red in urine.

6. Inject ADH 2 U into the marginal ear vein. Observe the change of urine volume.

[Precautions]

1. Feed the rabbit with adequate water before the experiment in order to increase the basal urine volume.

2. Conduct the experiment in sequential steps. Don't perform the next step until the former is completed.

3. Extract drugs with a syringe and don't mix up any of the drugs.

4. Use the scalp venous indwelling needle for the injection except for the anesthesia.

[Questions]

1. What happens to the urine volume in the rabbit after intravenous injection of 20 ml saline? Explain the mechanism for it.

2. What precautions should be taken in this experiment?

(Li Shumin)

实验九　心血管运动的神经体液调节

【实验目的】　学习哺乳类动物动脉血压的直接测量法；观察神经、体液因素对动脉血压的影响，从而了解心脏和血管活动的神经体液调节机制。

【实验原理】　颈动脉窦-主动脉弓压力感受性反射（减压反射）是维持动脉血压恒定的重要神经调节机制。当动脉血压升高时，血管壁张力增加，刺激压力感受器，减压反射增强，血压降低。当动脉血压降低时，压力感受器发放冲动减少，减压反射减弱，血压升高。人为改变反射弧中某一部分的活动，可引起动脉血压的变化。

肾上腺素和去甲肾上腺素是调节心血管运动的两个重要体液因素。肾上腺素可与 α 和 β 两类受体结合，使心脏收缩加强，心率加快，心输出量增加；其对血管的作用取决于血管平滑肌上两类受体分布的情况。去甲肾上腺素主要兴奋 α 受体，使血管收缩，外周阻力增加，血压升高，其对心脏的作用较肾上腺素弱。

【实验对象】　家兔

【实验用品】　BL-420 生物机能实验系统，哺乳类动物手术器械，兔手术台，保护电极，压力换能器，丝线，注射器，气管插管，动脉插管，动脉夹，25%氨基甲酸乙酯，1000 U/ml 肝素，10^{-4} mol/L 去甲肾上腺素

【实验步骤】

1. 麻醉、固定　家兔称重，25%氨基甲酸乙酯（4 ml/kg）耳缘静脉注射麻醉，家兔麻醉后，仰卧位固定于兔手术台上。

2. 颈部手术

（1）分离气管并插管。

（2）分离右侧减压神经、迷走神经以及双侧颈总动脉，分别穿线备用。

（3）耳缘静脉注入 1000 U/ml 肝素（1 ml/kg）进行全身肝素化，以防止凝血。

（4）左侧颈总动脉插管：结扎左侧颈总动脉远心端，近心端用动脉夹夹闭。用眼科剪在动脉上靠近结扎线处呈 45°角剪 "V" 形小口，约为管径的 1/3；然后将插管向心脏方向插入 2～4 cm，结扎固定；连接到 BL - 420 生物机能实验系统，小心缓慢打开动脉夹。

3. 调试仪器　点击菜单栏 "输入信号"，选择相应通道，点击 "压力" 信号和 "开始" 按钮，开始实验。

【观察项目】

1. 记录正常动脉血压曲线和数值，并观察其曲线波形特点。

2. 手持左侧颈总动脉上的头端结扎线，向心脏方向以 2～4 次/s 的频率，牵拉 5～10 s，观察动脉血压的变化。

3. 用动脉夹夹闭右侧颈总动脉约 15 s，观察动脉血压的变化。

4. 将减压神经置于保护电极上，以 3～5 V，30～70 Hz 连续脉冲进行刺激，观察动脉血压的变化；然后用两条丝线结扎减压神经，并从结扎线的中间剪断神经，用同样的刺激分别刺激其头端和心端，观察动脉血压的变化。

5. 用丝线结扎迷走神经，并在结扎线的头端剪断神经，刺激其心端，观察动脉血压的变化。

6. 耳缘静脉注射 10^{-4} mol/L 去甲肾上腺素 0.3 ml，观察动脉血压的变化。

【注意事项】

1. 在整个实验过程中，均需要保持动脉插管与颈总动脉于平行位置，防止动脉插管刺破动脉管壁。

2. 每完成一个项目必须待血压恢复后，才能进行下一项目的观察。

3. 实验结束后，先结扎颈总动脉，然后拔出动脉插管。

【思考题】

1. 支配心脏和血管的神经有哪些？各有什么作用？

2. 电刺激减压神经为什么分 3 次进行？其结果说明了什么？

3. 去甲肾上腺素和肾上腺素对血管的作用有何不同？

（张一兵）

Experiment 9　The neurohumoral regulation of the cardiovascular activities

〔**Experimental objectives**〕　To study the direct measurement of arterial blood pressure in mammals; to observe and analyze the effects of the neural and humoral factors on arterial blood pressure.

〔**Experimental principles**〕　Carotid sinus and aortic arch baroreceptor reflex（depressor reflex）is an important neural mechanism to maintain blood pressure. Increased tension of the vascular wall caused by high blood pressure can stimulate the baroreceptor, then the activities of depressor reflex increase and the blood pressure decreases. The decrease in blood pressure can lead to reduction in afferent impulse of baroreceptor, and then the activities of depressor reflex decrease and the blood pressure increases. If the activity of any part in reflex arc is changed artificially, the arterial blood pressure would change too.

Epinephrine and norepinephrine are two important humoral factors in regulating cardio-vascular activities. Epinephrine can bind with α and β receptor to cause the increase in heart contraction, heart rate and cardiac output. The effect of epinephrine on blood vessels depends on the distribution of two receptors on vascular smooth muscle. Norepinephrine mainly excites α receptor which causes the vasoconstriction and increase in peripheral resistance, and then blood pressure increases. The effect of norepinephrine on the heart is weaker than that of epinephrine.

[**Experimental object**] rabbit

[**Experimental materials**] BL – 420 system, surgical instruments for mammals, operation table for rabbit, shielded electrode, pressure transducer, thread, syringe, arterial clip, tracheal cannula, arterial cannula, 25% urethane, heparin solution (1000 U/ml), 10^{-4} mol/L norepinephrine

[**Experimental procedures**]

1. Anesthesia and fixation 25% ethylcarbamate (4 ml/kg) is injected into the marginal ear vein. Then the rabbit is fixed on the operating table in the supine body position after it has been anesthetized.

2. Operation on neck

(1) Separate the trachea and conduct intubation.

(2) Separate the right depressor nerve, vagus nerve and bilateral common carotid artery, and put threads under them for further use.

(3) Inject 1000 U/ml heparin solution (1 ml/kg) into the marginal ear vein to prevent from cruor.

(4) Left arterial intubation: Ligate the common carotid artery as near to the head end as is possible and clamp the artery near the heart end with an arterial clip. A "V"-shaped cut is made toward the heart end with sharp eye scissors between the knot and arterial clip at 45 degree angle. The cut is about one third diameter of the artery (cut as near as possible to the knot). Arterial cannula is inserted into the artery 2 – 4 cm from the incision toward the heart. Ligate and fix the cannula.

3. BL – 420 system adjustment Click "input signal" in menu bar and choose the "channel" and "pressure" signal, then click "start" button to start experiment.

[**Observations**]

1. Record the normal curve and the value of arterial blood pressure.

2. Softly drag the ligature thread of the left artery toward the direction of the heart for a few times, and observe the change of blood pressure.

3. Clamp the right common carotid artery for 15 s with an artery clip to stop blood flow, and observe the change of blood pressure.

4. Stimulate the right depressor nerve by a shielded electrode, and observe the change of blood pressure. The parameters of successive stimulus are as follows: intensity 3 – 5 V, fre-

quency 30 – 70 Hz. Ligate the depressor nerve with two threads and cut off the depressor nerve between two knots, then stimulate the distal end and the proximal end of depressor nerve respectively, and observe the change of blood pressure.

5. Ligate the right vagus nerve and cut off the nerve at the proximal end of the knot, stimulate the peripheral end with the intermediate intensity stimulus continuously (the parameters of stimulus are the same as above), and observe the change of blood pressure.

6. Inject 0.3 ml norepinephrine (10^{-4} mol/L) through the marginal ear vein, and observe the change of blood pressure.

[Precautions]

1. Keep the arterial cannula and the common carotid artery parallel to each other to avoid the artery being cut in the experiment.

2. Do not attempt to observe the next item until the blood pressure returns to normal upon the completion of the previous step.

3. When the experiment is finished, the common carotid artery is ligated at the proximal end firstly and then the arterial cannula is withdraw.

[Question]

1. Which nerves regulate the cardiovascular activity? What are their functions?

2. Why the depressor nerve is stimulated for three times? What do the results indicate?

3. What's the difference of effects on blood vessels between norepinephrine and epinephrine?

(Zhang Yibing)

实验十　反射时的测定与反射弧的分析

【实验目的】　观察常见的脊髓反射；理解反射弧各组成部分的功能及反射弧的完整性和反射活动的关系；学习反射时的测定方法。

【实验原理】　反射是在中枢神经系统的参与下，机体对刺激所做出的规律性应答，是神经活动的基本方式。反射的结构基础是反射弧。反射弧包括感受器、传入神经、神经中枢、传出神经和效应器五个部分。反射活动的完成有赖于反射弧的完整，如果反射弧中任一部分被破坏，反射将不能完成。脊髓是最低级的反射活动中枢，但脊髓的活动常受高位中枢的调节。为了观察脊髓反射，常将动物的高位中枢和脊髓之间的联系切断。只保留脊髓的动物称为脊动物，此时动物产生的各种反射则为脊髓反射，包括屈肌反射、搔爬反射和对侧伸肌反射等。从感受器接受刺激至机体出现反应所需要的时间称为反射时，即反射通过反射弧所用的时间。反射时的长短与反射经历突触的多少以及刺激强度有关。

【实验对象】　蛙或蟾蜍

【实验用品】　蛙类手术器械，蛙板，肌夹，培养皿，小烧杯，铁支架，纱布，滤纸片，秒表，0.5％硫酸溶液

【实验步骤】

1. 制备脊蟾蜍　左手持蟾蜍，食指按压头部前端，拇指按压背部，使头前俯。右手持

探针由头前端沿中线向尾端刺触，触及凹陷处即为枕骨大孔，将探针由此垂直刺入，再将探针尖端向头方刺入颅腔，左右搅动，破坏脑组织。

2. 固定　用肌夹夹住蟾蜍下颌，将其悬挂在铁支架上。

【观察项目】

1. 脊髓反射的观察

（1）屈肌反射　将蟾蜍左后肢的足趾尖浸入盛有 0.5％硫酸溶液的培养皿中，观察蟾蜍的屈肌反射。

（2）搔爬反射　将浸有 0.5％硫酸溶液的小滤纸片贴在蟾蜍背部或腹部的皮肤上，观察搔爬反射。

2. 反射时的测定

（1）屈肌反射时的测定　分别将蟾蜍左右后肢的最长趾浸入 0.5％硫酸溶液中（浸入 2～3 mm 为宜，浸入时间不要超过 10 s），同时用秒表记录从浸入硫酸溶液至出现屈肌反射所需要的时间，此为屈肌反射时。测定完成后迅速将该足趾上的硫酸用清水洗净，并用纱布擦干。上述步骤重复 3 次，求平均值。

（2）搔爬反射时的测定　将浸有 0.5％硫酸溶液的小滤纸片贴在蟾蜍背部或腹部的皮肤上，记录从刺激开始到发生反应的时间，重复 3 次，求平均值。

3. 反射弧的分析

（1）感受器损伤后的反应　在左后肢踝关节上方做一环形皮肤切口，在切口下方将足部皮肤剥去，用硫酸刺激被剥掉皮肤的趾端，观察机体的反应。

（2）神经损伤后的反应　取下蟾蜍，将右侧大腿背部皮肤剪开，沿着坐骨神经沟分离出坐骨神经并将其剪断，用硫酸刺激右侧趾尖，观察机体的反应。

（3）中枢损伤后的反应　取另一只蟾蜍捣毁脑组织，观察屈肌反射和搔爬反射。破坏蟾蜍脊髓后，重复观察项目 1，观察蟾蜍对刺激的不同反应。

【注意事项】

1. 刺激后立刻洗去硫酸以免损伤皮肤，并擦干水渍，防止硫酸被稀释。

2. 每次实验中，蟾蜍足趾浸入硫酸的范围应相同，以保持相同的刺激强度。

【思考题】

1. 为什么去掉趾部皮肤、切断坐骨神经和损坏脊髓以后反射会消失？

2. 反射时的长短受体内外哪些因素的影响？

（张　田）

Experiment 10　Measurement of reflex time and analysis of reflex arc

［**Experimental objectives**］　To observe several common spinal reflexes; to understand the functions of each component of reflex arc and the correlations between the integrity of reflex arc and reflex activity; to learn the measurement of reflex time.

［**Experimental principles**］　The reflex is the response process of the organism for stimulation in the participation of central nervous system, which is the basic way of neural regulation. The foundation of reflex activity is reflex arc. The components of a reflex arc include receptor, afferent pathway, nerve centre, efferent pathway and effector. The completion of a reflex activity relies on structural and functional integrity of reflex arc. If any part of the reflex arc is destroyed, reflex activities can not complete. The spinal cord is the lowest nervous centrum of many reflex activities. But the activities of spinal cord are regulated by superior centrum. In order to observe spinal reflex, the connection of the spinal cord and the brain are often cut off. This kind of animal is called spinal animal. Their reflex activities are pure spinal reflex including flexor reflex, scratching reflex, crossed extensor reflex and so on. The time period from stimulating receptor to the appearance of reflex is called reflex time. The length of reflex time is related with the number of synapse. and stimulus intensity.

[**Experimental object**]　toad or frog

[**Experimental materials**]　frog operating instruments, frog board, muscle clamp, culture dish, little beaker, iron stand, filter paper, gauze, stopwatch, 0.5% sulphuric acid

[**Experimental procedures**]

1. Preparation of spinal toad　Hold a toad with the left hand, press the front part of its head with forefinger and press its back with the thumb, make its head forward. Hold the probe with the right hand and move the probe down along the midline until the end of the skull. Prick the skin vertically at the hole of occipital bone, and then insert the probe pin into the cranial cavity and destroy the brain.

2. Fixation　Clip the toad's jaw with a muscle clamp and hang the toad on iron stand. Start the experiment after a while.

[**Observations**]

1. Observation of spinal reflex

(1) Flexor reflex: Immerse the skin on the left tiptoe of the toad hindlimb into 0.5% sulphuric acid in a culture dish, observe flexor reflex of the toad. Clean the skin with water.

(2) Scratching reflex: Stick a piece of filter paper which has been soaked in 0.5% sulphuric acid on the toad's abdomen, and observe scratching reflex of the toad. Clean the skin with water.

2. Measurement of the reflex time

(1) Flexor reflex time: Put some 0.5% sulphuric acid in the culture dish. Immerse the longest toe on the left and right hind leg in the culture dish respectively (2 – 3 mm in depth, not longer than 10 s). Record the time from the toe placed into sulfuric acid to the appearance of flexor reflex (the time between stimulus and response occurrence), which is flexor reflex time. Clean the skin with water and dry it with a piece of gauze. Repeat the above procedures for 3 times and then calculate the average time.

(2) Scratching reflex time: Stick a piece of filter paper which has been soaked in 0.5% sulphuric acid on the toad's abdomen, record the time between stimulus and response. Clean the sulfuric acid solution with water. Repeat the above procedures for 3 times and then calculate the average time.

3. Analysis of reflex arc

(1) Response of the toad to receptor injury: Cut a circle incision of its skin up the ankle joint of the left hind leg, peel off the skin of the lower limb, then stimulate its toe with 0.5% sulphuric acid, and observe the response of the toad.

(2) Response of the toad to nerve injury: Take down the toad. Cut a circle incision on the right thigh skin. Separate the sciatic nerve from the sciatic nerve ditch (between biceps femoris and semimembranosus) of the right leg and cut it off, then stimulate its toe skin with 0.5% sulphuric acid, and observe the response of the toad.

(3) Response of toad to nerve centre injury: Fetch another toad and destroy the brain according to the above method. Observe the flexor reflex and scratching reflex again. After the appearance of the reflex, push the probe down the vertebral canal and rotate the probe to destroy the spinal cord. Repeat observation step 1 and observe the different responses of the toad.

[**Precautions**]

1. Eliminate the sulfuric acid immediately with water after you finish each step, in order to avoid damaging the skin. And then wipe the water to prevent diluting sulphuric acid.

2. The dipping depth in sulfuric acid should be the same in order to maintain the same stimulus intensity.

[**Questions**]

1. Why does the reflex disappear when we peel off the skin, cut the sciatic nerve and destroy the spinal cord?

2. What are the main factors of that affect the length of reflex time in vivo and in vitro?

(Zhang Tian)

实验十一　给药剂量和给药途径对药物作用的影响

一、给药剂量对药物作用的影响

【实验目的】　观察药物的不同剂量对药物作用的影响。

【实验原理】　药理效应与剂量在一定范围内成正比，这就是量效关系。随着药物剂量的增加，药理效应也逐渐增强。水合氯醛为镇静催眠药，小剂量表现为镇静和嗜睡，随着剂量的加大表现为催眠、麻醉甚至死亡。

【实验对象】　小白鼠，体重 18～22 g，雌雄均可

【实验用品】　1%及 10%水合氯醛溶液，电子秤，注射器，针头，鼠笼

【实验步骤与观察项目】

1. 动物选择：取小白鼠 2 只，称重并编号，放入鼠笼内，观察正常活动。

2. 动物给药与结果观察：两鼠分别腹腔注射 1%及 10%水合氯醛溶液 0.1 ml/10 g 体重，置于鼠笼内，观察并记录给药后小鼠的反应及反应出现的时间。将实验结果填入表 4-3中。

表 4 - 3 给药剂量对药物作用的影响
表 4 - 3 给药剂量对药物作用的影响
Tab. 4 - 3 Influence of administration dose on drug effect of chloral hydrate

编号 Number	体重 Weight	药物用量 Dose	用药后反应 Reaction
1			
2			

【注意事项】

1. 腹腔注射过程中要确保药物注入腹腔。

2. 比较两小鼠所出现反应的严重程度。

【思考题】

1. 不同剂量的水合氯醛对小白鼠的作用有何不同?

2. 药物剂量和作用的关系对临床用药有何意义?

二、给药途径对药物作用的影响

【实验目的】 观察不同给药途径对药物作用的影响。

【实验原理】 不同给药途径有不同的药物吸收过程和特点,故药理效应也不同。常用的给药途径有口服、静脉注射、肌内注射、皮下注射等,给药途径不同药物产生的效应强度也有差别。硫酸镁为抗惊厥药,口服给药有泻下和利胆的作用,注射给药有抗惊厥作用。

【实验对象】 小白鼠,体重 $18 \sim 22$ g,雌雄均可

【实验用品】 10% 硫酸镁溶液,电子秤,注射器,针头,鼠笼

【实验步骤与观察项目】

1. 动物选择:小白鼠 2 只,称重后分别作标记,观察正常活动情况。

2. 动物给药与结果观察:一鼠灌胃 10% $MgSO_4$ 溶液 0.2 ml/10 g 体重,另一鼠皮下注射等量 10% $MgSO_4$ 溶液。分别置于鼠笼中,观察并记录给药后小鼠的反应及反应出现的时间。将实验结果填入表 4 - 4 中。

表 4 - 4 给药途径对药物作用的影响
Tab. 4 - 4 Influence of administration route on drug action of magnesium sulfate

小鼠编号 Number	体重 Weight	药物用量 Dose	给药途径 Route	用药后反应 Reaction
1				
2				

【注意事项】

1. 灌胃给药及皮下注射给药要熟练。

2. 注射药物后作用发生较快,需注意观察动物反应。

【思考题】

1. 硫酸镁经不同给药途径对小白鼠的作用有何不同?

2. 不同给药途径对药物作用产生差异的原因？

（张博男）

Experiment 11 The influence of dose and administration route on drug effect

Part 1. The influence of administration dose on drug effect

〔**Experimental objective**〕 To observe the influence of administration dose on drug effect.

〔**Experimental principles**〕 Pharmacological effect is proportional to dose within a certain range and this is known as the dose-effect relationship. With the increase of drug dose, the pharmacological effect gradually increases. Chloral hydrate is a sedative hypnotic. Sedation and drowsiness appear with low doses, then with the increase of dose, this drug produces a hypnotic state, anesthesia and death.

〔**Experimental object**〕 mouse, 18 – 22 g, male or female

〔**Experimental materials**〕 1% and 10% chloral hydrate solution, electronic balance, syringe, needle and mouse cage

〔**Experimental procedures and Observations**〕

1. Animal selection Select two mice, weight and mark them and observe the normal movements.

2. Drug administration The two mice are to receive intraperitoneal injection with 1% and 10% chloral hydrate 0.1 ml/10 g, respectively.

3. Outcome observation Observe the changes of the movements and whether the body-righting reflex has disappeared. Record the changes of the symptoms between the time of administration to the time when pharmacological effect appears. Fill the record in the Tab. 4 – 3 and compare the difference between the two mice.

〔**Precautions**〕

1. Make sure the drug is injected into the abdominal cavity through intraperitoneal injection.

2. Compare the extent of reaction in the two mice.

〔**Questions**〕

1. What is the different effect of chloral hydrate in different doses on mice?

2. What is the signifcance of the correlations between the drug dose and effect for guidance of taking medicine in clinic?

Part 2. The influence of administration route on drug effect

〔**Experimental objective**〕 To observe the influence of administration route on drug effect.

〔**Experimental principles**〕 The drug absorptive process and characteristics vary through different routes of drug administration; therefore the corresponding pharmacological effect is different. Some common administration routes such as oral administration, intravenous injection, intramuscular injection and subcutaneous injection. Different administrative route may appear different drug effect. For instance, as an anticonvulsant, magnesium sulfate produces diarrhoea and cholagogue when administrated through oral route and appears anticonvulsant effect when administrated through injection route.

〔**Experimental object**〕 mouse, 18 - 22 g, male or female

〔**Experimental materials**〕 10% magnesium sulfate solution, electronic balance, syringe, needle, mouse cage

〔**Experimental procedures and Observations**〕

1. Animal selection　Weigh and mark the two mice and observe the normal movements.

2. Drug administration　One mouse is to receive subcutaneous injection with 10% magnesium sulfate 0. 2 ml/10 g and the other is to receive oral administration with 10% magnesium sulfate 0. 2 ml/10 g.

3. Outcome observation　Observe the changes of the movement and whether the body-righting reflex disappears. Record the changes of the symptoms from the time of administration to the time when pharmacological effect appears. Fill the record in the Tab. 4 - 4 and compare the difference of the two mice.

〔**Precautions**〕

1. Make sure subcutaneous injection and oral administration are performed successfully.

2. Closely monitor the animal reaction because the effect of injection administration appears rapidly.

〔**Questions**〕

1. What is the difference in mouse reactions between different administration routes of magnesium sulfate?

2. Why is the pharmacological effect different between administration routes?

(Zhang Bonan)

实验十二　镇痛药物实验

【实验目的】　掌握不同类型镇痛药的镇痛机制；比较镇痛药和解热镇痛药在镇痛作用上的差别；了解测定药物的镇痛强度常用的实验方法。

【实验原理】　疼痛是一种因组织损伤或潜在的组织损伤而产生的痛苦感觉，常伴有不愉快的情绪反应。它既是机体的一种保护性机制，提醒机体避开这种伤害，也是许多疾病的常见症状。根据疼痛的发生部位的不同可分为躯体痛、内脏痛和神经痛三种类型。缓解疼痛的药物主要包括阿片类镇痛药和解热镇痛药。阿片类镇痛药的镇痛部位在中枢，通过激动阿片受体，模拟内源性阿片肽，阻断痛觉冲动的传导通路而产生镇痛作用。此类药物镇痛作用强大，对多种剧痛有效。解热镇痛药的镇痛部位在外周，通过抑制环氧酶（前列腺素合成酶），使前列腺素（PG）合成减少而产生镇痛作用。研究镇痛药的实验方法通常通过给予动物一定的伤害性刺激，观察其逃避或防御反应。常用的镇痛药物实验方法有机械刺激法、热刺激法、电刺激法、化学物质刺激法。

一、热板法测定药物的镇痛作用

【实验对象】　小鼠（雌性，体重 18～22 g）

【实验用品】　0.4％曲马多溶液，3.6％赖氨匹林溶液，生理盐水，热板仪，小鼠笼，1 ml 注射器，针头，烧杯，电子秤

【实验步骤与观察项目】

1. 动物筛选　取体重 18～22 g 的小鼠，置于热板仪上（温度为 55℃±0.5 ℃），测定各小鼠正常的痛阈值，观测指标为小鼠舔后足。痛阈值在 5 ～30 s 之间的为合格小鼠。每一实验组选出 3 只合格小鼠。

2. 分组给药　A 鼠腹腔注射 0.4％曲马多，给药量按 0.1 ml/10 g；B 鼠腹腔注射 3.6％赖氨匹林溶液 0.1 ml/10 g；C 鼠腹腔注射生理盐水 0.1 ml/10 g。

3. 测定给药后痛阈值　各小鼠在给药后 15 min 再测一次痛阈值。如果小鼠 60 s 还无痛反应，则按 60 s 计算。

4. 汇总结果　汇总整个实验室的实验结果，并填入表 4 - 5。

按以下公式计算痛阈提高百分率：痛阈提高百分率（TB）＝（药后痛阈值－药前痛阈值）/药前痛阈值×100％（若药后痛阈减去药前痛阈为负数，则按零计算）

表 4 - 5　曲马多与赖氨匹林镇痛作用比较

Tab. 4 - 5　Contrast of the analgesic effect of tramadol and lysine-acetylsalicylate

组别 Group	A 小鼠痛阈值（s）Pain threshold of mouse A			B 小鼠痛阈值（s）Pain threshold of mouse B			C 小鼠痛阈值（s）Pain threshold of mouse C		
	药前 Before	药后 After	TB（％）	药前 Before	药后 After	TB（％）	药前 Before	药后 After	TB（％）
1									
2									
3									
4									
5									
6									
平均值 Mean									

【注意事项】

1. 应选用雌性小鼠，不能使用雄性小鼠（因为雄性小鼠受热后阴囊下坠，阴囊皮肤对

疼痛太敏感）。

2. 只有舔后足才能作为疼痛的观察指标。

3. 测定痛反应时，一旦出现典型的疼痛症状，即应立即移开热板；60 s 还无痛反应时也应立即移开热板，以免烫伤。

二、扭体法测定药物的镇痛作用

【实验对象】 小鼠（雌雄均可）

【实验用品】 0.4％曲马多溶液，3.6％赖氨匹林溶液，0.6％醋酸，生理盐水，小鼠笼，1 ml 注射器，针头，烧杯，电子秤

【实验步骤与观察项目】

1. 分组 取小鼠 6 只，随机分为 3 组。

2. 给药 A 组鼠腹腔注射 0.4％曲马多，给药量按 0.1 ml/10 g；B 组鼠腹腔注射 3.6％赖氨匹林溶液 0.1 ml/10 g；C 组鼠腹腔注射生理盐水 0.1 ml/10 g。

3. 给醋酸 15 min 后，各小鼠再分别腹腔注射 0.6％醋酸溶液 0.2 ml/只。

4. 观察现象 观察给醋酸溶液 20 min 内各组小鼠扭体反应动物数及扭体反应的次数，并将结果填入表 4 - 6。

5. 汇总结果 汇总全班实验结果，并按以下公式计算镇痛百分率：镇痛百分率＝（实验组无扭体反应动物数-对照组无扭体反应动物数）/实验组动物数×100％

表 4 - 6 曲马多与赖氨匹林镇痛作用比较
Tab. 4 - 6 Contrast of the analgesic effect of tramadol and lysine-acetylsalicylate

组别 Group	实验组无扭体反应动物数 Number of the mice without writhing in experimental group		对照组无扭体反应动物数 Number of mice without writhing in control group
	曲马多组 Tramadol group	赖氨匹林组 L-ASA group	
1			
2			
3			
4			
5			
6			
平均值 Mean			

【注意事项】

1. 醋酸溶液需临时配制，如放置过久，作用明显减弱。

2. 化学物质刺激法应在室温 20 ℃左右进行，温度过低或过高对扭体反应有影响。

3. 小鼠体重应在 22～26 g，因为体重过轻，扭体反应出现率低。

【思考题】

1. 曲马多和赖氨匹林哪个药物镇痛效果更好？为什么？

2. 常用的镇痛药物实验方法有哪些？

（王树华）

Experiment 12　Action of analgesic drugs

[Experimental objectives] To master analgesia mechanism of different types of analgesics; to compare the difference of analgesic effect between analgesics and antipyretic analgesics; to understand general experimental methods that determine analgesia intension of analgesics.

[Experimental principles] Pain is a suffering sensation due to actual or potential tissue damage, often accompanied with an unpleasant emotional response. It is one kind of protective mechanism that alerts a person to avoid injury; meanwhile, it is also a common symptom for many diseases. Depending on the site of the occurrence, pain can be divided into three types: somatic pain, visceral pain and neuropathic pain. Drugs for pain relief mainly include Opioid Analgesics and antipyretic analgesics. The action site of Opioid Analgesics is at central nervous system (CNS); by activating the opioid receptors, they can simulate endogenous opioid peptides, block the conduction pathways of painful impulse and thus generate analgesic effect. Opioids are powerful pain-relieving substances and they are effective in treating a variety of acute pains. In contrast, antipyretic analgesics target at peripheral nervous system (PNS) and generate analgesic effect by inhibiting epoxidase (prostaglandin synthetase) and making prostaglandin (PG) synthesis decrease. Experimental methods for analgesics study usually involve giving the animal some kind of noxious stimulation to observe its escape or defensive reactions. Commonly used experimental methods include mechanical stimulation, thermal stimulation, electrical stimulation and chemical stimulation.

Part 1. Analgesic effect of drugs by hot plate test

[Experimental object]　female mouse (18 – 22 g)

[Experimental materials]　0.4% tramadol, 3.6% lysine-acetylsalicylate solution (L – ASA, a Soluble Salt of Aspirin), normal saline, electric hot plate, mouse cage, 1 ml syringes, needles, beakers, balance

[Experimental procedures and observations]

1. Animals selection: Set the temperature at $55^{\circ}\text{C} \pm 0.5^{\circ}\text{C}$ and place a mouse on the hot plate. Then turn on the stopwatch and record the time, and observe the mouse's reaction to thermal stimulation. The pain reaction is identified as licking its own hind paw, and as such the mouse should be taken off the hot plate when it licks itself. The mouse can be used to do the test when its pain reaction happens in 5 – 30 s. The pain reaction time is used as the normal pain threshold before drug treatment. Each group includes 3 eligible mice whose pain threshold is 5 – 30 s.

2. Drug administration by group: Mouse A is treated with 0.4% tramadol by intraperitoneal injection, 0.1 ml/10 g. Mouse B is treated with 3.6% L – ASA by intraperitoneal injection, 0.1 ml/10 g. Mouse C is given normal saline by intraperitoneal injection, 0.1 ml /10 g.

3. To measure the pain threshold after treatment: After treatment, all mice have their

pain threshold determined after 15 min according to the method above. If the mouse fails to lick its hind paw itself with in 60 s, its pain threshold is regarded as 60 s.

4. Collection of the experimental results: Collect the experimental results of the whole laboratory class and fill in the following Tab. 4 - 5.

Calculate the increased percentage of pain threshold of the mouse according to the following formula: The analgesia percentage of drug = (pain threshold after administration – pain threshold before administration) /pain threshold before administration×100%.

[Precautions]

1. Female mice should be selected for this experiment. Male mice can't be used for this experiment, because their scrotum will droop down to the hot plate and cause the mouse to jump and influence the experimental result judgement.

2. Licking hind paw is the unique observational indicator of pain.

3. When measuring pain reactions, the mouse must be moved from the hot plate when appearing typical pain symptom; If the mouse fail to lick hind paw itself within 60 s, the mouse immediately in order to avoid being burnt.

Part 2. Analgesic effect of drugs by writing test

[Experimental object]　mouse (female or male)

[Experimental materials]　0.4% tramadol, 3.6% L-ASA, 0.6% Acetic acid solution, normal saline, mouse cage, 1 ml syringes, needles, beakers, balance

[Experimental procedures and observations]

1. Group the mice　Six mice are divided into 3 groups randomly.

2. Give the following drugs to mice　Mice in group A are treated with 0.4% tramadol by intraperitoneal injection, 0.1 ml/10 g. Mice in group B are treated with 3.6% L-ASA by intraperitoneal injection, 0.1 ml/10 g. Mice in group C are treated with normal saline by intraperitoneal injection, 0.1 ml /10 g.

3. Give acetic acid　After 15 min, each mouse is rendered with 0.2 ml 0.6% acetic acid through intraperitoneal injection, respectively.

4. Observe phenomenon　In 20 min, record the number of writhing mice and the writhing frequency, and fill in the following Tab. 4 - 6.

5. Collect the experimental results　Collect the results of the whole laboratory class and calculate the analgesia percentage of drug according to the following formula: The analgesia percentage of drug = (animal number of no writhing in experimental group-animal number of no writhing in control group)/ animal number in experimental group×100%.

[Precautions]

1. Acetic acid solution must be newly prepared, because its effect will be weakened markedly over time.

2. Keep the room temperature constant (20 ℃), because the room temperature (high or low) will affect the writhing reactions.

3. Body weight of the experimental mice should be between 22 to 26 g, because the writhing frequency will decrease if underweight.

[**Questions**]

1. Which drug produces better analgesia effect between tramadol and lysine-acetylsalicylate? Why?

2. What are the commonly used analgesic experiment methods?

(Wang Shuhua)

实验十三　pH 对药物排泄的影响

【实验目的】　掌握尿液 pH 的改变对水杨酸钠排泄的影响，并解释其原理。

【实验原理】　药物主要以分子状态经生物膜转运。绝大多数的药物呈弱酸性或弱碱性，尿液的 PH 值会影响药物的解离度，从而影响药物在肾小管的重吸收，最终影响药物的排泄。弱酸性药物在碱性尿液中主要以离子状态存在，所以重吸收少，排泄多，在酸性尿液中正相反；反之，弱碱性药物在碱性尿液中重吸收多，排泄少，在酸性尿液中正相反。显色原理：水杨酸钠与三氯化铁反应可生成一种紫色络合物。生成的络合物颜色越深，说明参与反应的水杨酸钠浓度越高。再通过与标准管比色，可确定尿液中排出的水杨酸钠的大致浓度。

【实验对象】　大鼠，体重 220～260 g，雌雄皆可

【实验用品】　10%氯化铵溶液，12%碳酸氢钠溶液，10%水杨酸钠溶液，呋塞米，10%水合氯醛溶液，酸性蒸馏水，1%三氯化铁溶液，大鼠灌胃器，刻度试管，试管架，刻度吸管，洗耳球，注射器，针头，pH 试纸，棉线，蛙板，大鼠笼，标准管，烧杯

【实验步骤与观察项目】

1. 制造酸、碱环境　禁食 12 h 大鼠 6 只，每组 3 只。称重，3 只灌胃 12%碳酸氢钠溶液 0.5 ml/100 g，3 只灌胃 10%氯化铵溶液 0.5 ml/100 g。

2. 灌水　30 min 后，灌胃饮用水 2 ml/100 g。

3. 给药　灌水后 15 min，每只大鼠腹腔注射 10%水杨酸钠溶液 0.3 ml/100 g。随后腹腔注射 10%水合氯醛溶液 0.2 ml/100 g。

4. 注射速尿　10 min 后，腹腔注射呋塞米，每只 0.5 ml。

5. 收集尿液　将大鼠仰卧固定于操作台上，取刻度试管置尿道口收集注射水杨酸钠后 40 min 内的尿液，记录总尿量（ml）。

6. pH 测定　取适量尿液，用 pH 试纸测定 pH 值。

7. 显色　取 1 ml 尿液，加 2 ml 酸性蒸馏水，再加 1%三氯化铁溶液 0.5 ml，摇匀显色，与标准管比较。对照附表，确定尿液中排泄出水杨酸钠的浓度（mg/ml）。

8. 计算　计算尿液中排泄水杨酸钠的剂量（mg），将结果填入表 4-7。

表 4-7　尿液 pH 的改变对水杨酸钠排泄的影响

Tab. 4-7　Influence of urinary pH on sodium salicylate excretion

组别 Group	总尿量（ml）Total urine volume	尿液 pH Urinary pH	尿药浓度（mg/ml）Drug concentration	总排药量（mg）Total excreted drug
碳酸氢钠组 NH₄Cl				
1				
2				
3				
平均值 Mean				
氯化铵组 NaHCO₃				
1				
2				
3				
平均值 Mean				

附　表（Attached table）

试管编号 Tuber number	1	2	3	4	5	6	7
浓度（mg/ml）Concentration	0.8	0.4	0.2	0.15	0.1	0.05	0.025

【注意事项】

1. 灌胃给药要小心仔细操作，防止误入气管。

2. 给药剂量和时间要准确。

3. 酸、碱药物不要混淆。

4. 尿液收集时间要准确。

【思考题】

1. 水杨酸钠呈酸性还是碱性？给予碳酸氢钠和氯化铵后尿液中水杨酸钠排泄有何不同？原因是什么？

2. 通过改变尿液的 pH 对临床用药有何指导意义？

（储金秀）

Experiment 13　Influence of urinary pH on drug excretion

〔**Experimental objectives**〕　To observe the influence of altering urinary pH on sodium salicylate excretion and to explain the principles.

〔**Experimental principles**〕　Drugs primarily pass across cell membranes through molecular diffusion and transport. As most drugs are either weak acids or weak bases, so the pH of the urine will influence the degree of dissociation of a drug, which thereby influences the renal tabular reabsorption of the drug and ultimately influences its excretion. Weakly acidic drugs tend to exist in the ionized form when exposed to the basic urine, so they are less reabsorbed and more excreted, and vice verse when they are exposed to the acidic urine. On the

71

contrary, weak basic drugs are more reabsorbed and less excreted when exposed to the basic urine, and have opposite results when exposed to the acidic urine. Principle of the chromogenic reaction: A purple chelate is produced by reaction of sodium salicylate ($C_7H_5NaO_3$) with $FeCl_3$. The darker the color looks, the more chelate is produced. This indicates that more $C_7H_5NaO_3$ has been excreted. The concentration of $C_7H_5NaO_3$ excreted from the urine can be read roughly by referring to the standard tubes.

[Experimental object]　rat, weight (220 - 260) g, male or female

[Experimental materials]　10% NH_4Cl, 12% $NaHCO_3$, 10% $C_7H_5NaO_3$, Furosemide, 10% chloral hydrate, acid distilled water, 1% $FeCl_3$, intragastric injection needles, graduated test tubes, test tube stand, graduated pipettes, rubber pipette bulb, syringes and needles, pH indicator paper, cotton thread, animal operating-table, rat cage, standard tubes, beaker

[Experimental procedures and observational items]

1. Change of the urinary pH　Select 6 rats with fasting 12 hours, and divide them into 2 groups. Weigh the rat, and intragastrically inject 10% NH_4Cl or 12% $NaHCO_3$ 0.5 ml/100 g.

2. Water lavage　30 min later, intragastrically inject water 2 ml/100 g.

3. Injection of $C_7H_5NaO_3$　15 min later, intraperitoneally inject $C_7H_5NaO_3$ 0.3 ml/100 g, followed by 10% chloral hydrate 0.2 ml/100 g through intraperitoneal injection.

4. Injection of Furosemide　10 min later, intraperitoneally inject Furosemide 0.5 ml to each rat.

5. Collection of urine　Fix the rat onto the operating table in the supine position, collect the urine into a graduated test tube for 40 min, and record the total volume of urine (ml).

6. pH measurement　Measure the urinary pH with pH indicator paper.

7. Chromogenic reaction　Add acid distilled water 2.0 ml to 1.0 ml of urine, followed by $FeCl_3$ 0.5 ml, shake the mixture and compare it with the standard tubes. Read the concentration of $C_7H_5NaO_3$ (mg/ml) in the urine according to the attached table.

8. Calculation　Calculate the excretion of sodium salicylate in the urine (mg) and fill the results in the Tab. 4 - 7.

[Precautions]

1. Be careful during intragastric administration, and avoid injection into the trachea.

2. The dosages administered and time interval should be accurate.

3. Don't mix up the drugs and reagents.

4. The collecting time should be accurate.

[Questions]

1. Is $C_7H_5NaO_3$ acidic or basic? How does NH_4Cl or $NaHCO_3$ influence the excretion of $C_7H_5NaO_3$? Why?

2. What is the clinical significance of regulating the excretion of drugs by altering urinary pH?

(Chu Jinxiu)

实验十四　有机磷中毒及解救

【实验目的】　观察有机磷药物中毒的症状及机制。观察阿托品和解磷定对有机磷中毒的解救作用及机制。

【实验原理】　有机磷酸酯属于难逆性胆碱酯酶抑制药，进入机体内可抑制胆碱酯酶的活性，使胆碱酯酶水解乙酰胆碱（Acetylcholine，ACh）减少，造成 ACh 在体内大量堆积而产生一系列中毒症状（包括 M 样、N 样及 CNS 症状）。阿托品为 M 受体阻断药，能迅速缓解 M 症状及部分中枢症状，解磷定为胆碱酯酶复活药，可恢复胆碱酯酶水解 ACh 的活性，并可直接与游离的有机磷结合成无毒的物质，从尿中排除，从而解除有机磷中毒。

【实验对象】　家兔

【实验用品】　0.5% 阿托品溶液，10% 敌百虫溶液（Dipterex），2.5% 解磷定；5 ml 注射器 3 支，兔固定箱，瞳孔尺，刀片，滤纸，棉花，止血夹一个

【实验步骤与实验项目】

1. 家兔称重　取家兔，称重，固定于兔盒中。观察下列指标：瞳孔大小、唾液分泌、大小便、肌张力及有无肌震颤等，分别加以记录。

2. 注射有机磷　腹腔注射有机磷农药：10% Dipterex 3 ml/kg。注意给药后家兔上述生理指标的变化，加以记录。

3. 中毒解救　中毒症状明显时，立即给家兔耳缘静脉静脉注射 0.5% 阿托品 0.4 ml/kg，再检查各项生理指标，待瞳孔散大，唾液明显减少后，立即耳缘静脉注射 2.5% 解磷定 1 ml/kg，观察中毒消除症状。

表 4 - 8　家兔有机磷中毒和解救后表现

Tab. 4 - 8　Manifestations of organophosphorus poisoning in rabbits

观察时间 Time	瞳孔大小（cm） Pupil size	唾液分泌 Saliva secretion	大小便 Urine and faeces	肌张力 Muscle tension	肌震颤 Muscular tremor
正常 Normal					
给敌百虫后 Post-admin of Dipterex					
给阿托品后 Post-admin of Atropine					
给解磷定后 Post-admin of Pralidoxime					

【注意事项】

1. 敌百虫属于有毒物质，可以通过皮肤吸收。实验过程中手接触到敌百虫后，立即用清水洗去。不能用碱性肥皂进行洗涤，因为敌百虫在碱性环境下会变成敌敌畏，毒性增加。

2. 瞳孔大小受光线的影响，测量瞳孔时应光线适中，每次均于同一光线下测。

3. 本试验系为分析阿托品和解磷定的解毒机制而设计。在临床实际应用中，需将阿托

品与解磷定配合应用，才能获得最佳解毒效果。

【思考题】

1. 有机磷农药中毒的机制是什么？可出现哪些症状？

2. 阿托品和解磷定的解毒机制各是什么？本实验解毒时为什么先注射阿托品，后注射解磷定？

（勾向博）

Experiment 14　Acute intoxication of organophosphate compound and its treatment

[**Experimental objectives**]　To observe the symptoms of organophosphorus poisoning and analyze the mechanism; to observe the rescue effect of atropine and pralidoxime to this condition and investigate the mechanism.

[**Experimental principles**]　Organophosphate is an irreversible cholinesterase inhibitor, which can inhibit cholinesterase activity, upon entering the body and decrease the hydrolysis of acetylcholine by cholinesterase, resulting in large accumulation of acetylcholine in the body to cause symptoms of poisoning such as muscarinic, nicotinic and CNS symptoms. As a muscarinic receptor antagonist, atropine can alleviate muscarinic and some CNS symptoms; in addition, pralidoxime is a cholinesterase reactivator which can recover cholinesterase activity as well as combine with free organophosphate to form non-toxic substances that will be excreted through urine.

[**Experimental object**]　rabbit

[**Experimental materials**]　0.5% Atropine solution, 10% Dipterex solution, 2.5% pralidoxime solution, syringes (5 ml), pupil ruler, blade, filter paper, cotton, hemostatic clamp, rabbit restraint box

[**Experimental procedure and observational items**]

1. Rabbit weighing　Weigh the rabbit and fix it in a rabbit restraint box. Observe and record the following indicators: pupil size, saliva, urine and faeces, muscle tension and presence of muscular tremors.

2. Injection of dipterex　The rabbit is given Dipterex (3 ml/kg) through intraperitoneal injection and the foresaid indicators are observed and recorded.

3. The treatment of acute intoxication　The rabbit receives atropine (0.4 ml/kg) when the symptoms of poisoning become apparent; at the same time we should record the above indicators. Pralidoxime (1 ml/kg) will be injected by intravenous injection when the pupils of eyes dilates and the saliva decreases and the indicators should also be recorded.

[**Precautions**]

1. Dipterex is a powerful toxicant which can be absorbed via skin. Wash your hands with water immediately if they are closed to Dipterex during the experiment. Alkali soaps are not allowed to be used because dipterex will transform to dichlorvos that has an even

74

stronger toxicity.

2. As the size of pupil is influenced by light, the rabbit should be kept under the same moderate light during each measurement.

3. This experiment is designed to analyze the mechanism of detoxication of atropine and pralidoxime. In clinical practice, the two drugs should be applied together to obtain optimal effect of detoxication.

[**Questions**]

1. What is the mechanism of organophosphate poisoning? What symptoms will appear when organophosphate poisoning occurs?

2. What are the respective mechanisms of detoxication of atropine and pralidoxime? Why should atropine be injected before pralidoxime in this experiment?

(Gou Xiangbo)

实验十五　药物半衰期测定

【实验目的】　用比色法测定磺胺甲噁唑（sulfamethoxazole，SMZ）的血药浓度并计算其半衰期。

【实验原理】　在治疗剂量下体内大多数药物按照一级动力学消除，一级动力学消除半衰期公式为 $t_{1/2} = 0.693/k_e$，k_e 为消除速率常数。此公式可转换成 $t_{1/2} = 0.301 (t_2 - t_1) / (\lg C_1 - \lg C_2)$。$C_1$、$C_2$ 表示药物在 t_1、t_2 时间的浓度。因此，在任意两时间点的药物浓度被测定，将能够求得 $t_{1/2}$。在本实验中，被测定的药物为磺胺甲噁唑，不同时间点的药物浓度通过比色法测定。

【实验对象】　家兔

【实验用品】　3%磺胺甲噁唑，7.5%三氯醋酸，0.5%亚硝酸钠，0.5%麝香草酚，草酸钾，0.5、1、2、5、10 ml 移液管，离心机，722 型分光光度计

【实验步骤与观察项目】

1. 给药前取血　取家兔一只称重，给药前从颈总动脉处取血 0.8 ml 置于放有草酸钾粉剂的小烧杯（1 号烧杯）中。

2. 给药及给药后取血　由耳缘静脉注射 3% 的 SMZ 溶液 1 ml/kg。给药后 5 min 和 35 min 各从颈总动脉取血约 0.8ml 于另两个放有草酸钾的小烧杯（2 号和 3 号烧杯）中，振摇后备用。

3. 沉淀蛋白　用 0.5 ml 移液管准确吸取上述兔血 0.4 ml 于离心管中。离心管中预先加 7.5%三氯醋酸 5.6 ml，用玻璃棒充分搅拌均匀，离心 1500 转，5 min，使血浆蛋白沉淀。

4. 重氮化和偶合反应　准确吸取离心管中之上清液 3 ml，依次加入 0.5%亚硝酸钠1 ml 和 0.5%麝香草酚溶液 2 ml 摇匀后，即可见深浅不同的橙色。

5. 比色测定　显色 15 min 后比色，以给药前为对照管，置于分光光度计（525 nm 波长）比色，得出给药后两管上清液的光密度值 X_1 和 X_2。根据回归方程 $C = (X + 0.0186) / 0.0011$，计算血药浓度 C_1 和 C_2。再根据公式 $t_{1/2} = 0.301 (t_2 - t_1) / (\lg C_1 - \lg C_2)$ 计算 $t_{1/2}$。将结果填入表 4-9。

表 4-9　给药后不同时间 SMZ 的光密度和血浆药物浓度
Tab. 4-9　Optical density and blood concentration of SMZ at different time points after administration

试管编号 Tube number		光密度（X）Optical density	血浆药物浓度（C）Concentration
给药后 5 min	5 min after administration	$X_1 =$	$C_1 =$
给药后 35 min	35 min after administration	$X_2 =$	$C_2 =$

计算半衰期 $t_{1/2}$。

【注意事项】

1. 用合适刻度的移液管吸取相应的溶液，不可混用。

2. 吸取上清液后，应按照顺序先加入亚硝酸钠，反应片刻后再加入麝香草酚，否则反应将不能正常进行。

3. 3 种样品应同时进行显色反应以保持显色时间一致。

【思考题】

1. 测定半衰期有何临床意义？

2. 简述影响半衰期的因素？

（白　静）

Experiment 15　Measurement of the half-life time of a drug

［**Experimental objectives**］　To determining the concentration of sulfamethoxazole (SMZ) by colorimetric method and calculate the half-life.

［**Experimental principles**］　Most drugs in the body are eliminated according to the first-order elimination kinetics, formula $t_{1/2} = 0.693/ke$, where ke is the elimination rate constant. This formula can be converted to $t_{1/2} = 0.301 (t_2 - t_1) / (lgC_1 - lgC_2)$, where C_1 and C_2 represent the concentrations of a drug at time t_1 and time t_2. Thus if the concentrations of a drug in blood plasma is measured at different times, the half-life time would be calculated. In this experiment, SMZ is the drug to be measured and the drug concentrations at different time points could be obtained by colorimetric method.

［**Experimental object**］　rabbit

［**Experimental materials**］　3% sulfamethoxazole (SMZ), 0.5% sodium nitrite, 0.5% thymol, 7.5% trichloroacetic acid, potassium oxalate powder, pipettes, centrifuge, spectrophotometer Model 722

［**Experimental procedures and observations**］

1. Blood drawing before administration　Take a rabbit, to measure its weight, collect about 0.8 ml of blood from its common carotid artery and place it in No. 1 small beaker in which some potassium oxalate powders has been placed beforehand.

2. Administration and blood drawing　The rabbit is given 3% SMZ (1.0 ml/kg) by intravenous injection in the marginal ear vein. Collect about 0.8 ml of blood respectively after 5 min and 35 min, and place them in No. 2 and No. 3 beakers, which also have had some po-

tassium oxalate powder placed inside before hand.

3. Protein precipitation   Draw 0. 4 ml of the above blood sample with 0. 5 ml pipette and place them in these three centrifuge tube，and shake slightly. 5. 6 ml of 7. 5% trichloro-acetic acid are pre-added into each tube. Centrifuge three tubes at 1500 rpm for 5 min.

4. Diazo and azo reaction   Draw 3 ml of supernatant from each tube and place them in another three numbered tubes，respectively. Add 1 ml of 0. 5% sodium nitrite into each tube and shake slightly. In addition，add 2 ml of 0. 5% thymol solution into each tube. Shake slightly again.

5. Colorimetric assay   After 15 min，read optical density of each tube on spectropho-tometer at 525 nm of wavelength. （When measuring allow the optical density of No. 1 tube equal to zero. So X_1 represents optical density of No. 2 tube and X_2 represents optical density of No. 3 tube.) Calculate the corresponding concentration value of C_1 and C_2 according to the following formula：$C = (X + 0.0186) / 0.0011$. Calculate $t_{1/2}$ by means of the following for-mula：$t_{1/2} = 0.301 (t_2 - t_1) / (lgC_1 - lgC_2)$.   Fill the experimental results in Tab. 4 - 9.

Calculate $t_{1/2}$.

[Precautions]

1. The pipettes with appropriate calibrations should be used to pipette corresponding so-lution. Do not mix them.

2. Sodium nitrite should be added in the supernatant first to allow time for reaction，and then the thymol is added.

3. The color reaction of three samples should begin simultaneously in order to make the color-developing time consistent.

[Questions]

1. What is the significance of measuring the half-life of a drug?

2. What are the factors that influence the half-life of a drug?

(Bai Jing)

实验十六   组胺和抗组胺药对离体肠平滑肌的影响

【实验目的】   观察不同剂量的组胺对豚鼠回肠平滑肌的收缩作用及苯海拉明对其作用的影响。

【实验原理】   组胺（Histamine）是广泛存在于组织的自身活性物质，其与靶细胞上组胺受体（H_1，H_2，H_3）结合，产生各种生物效应。H_1受体分布于各种平滑肌，豚鼠回肠平滑肌对其特别敏感，组胺作用可引起豚鼠回肠平滑肌明显收缩。竞争性拮抗药是指能与激动药受体可逆性结合，并且无内在活性的化合物，能使激动药的量-效反应曲线平行右移，但最大效应 Emax 保持不变。苯海拉明为组胺 H_1 受体竞争性拮抗药，能阻断组胺与 H_1 受体的结合，从而产生抗组胺作用。

【实验对象】   豚鼠，体重 200～300 g

【实验用品】   BL - 420 生物机能实验系统，计算机，张力传感器，保温式麦氏浴槽，超级恒温水浴，"L"形通气钩，高位吊瓶，量筒，烧杯，培养器，氧气瓶，外科剪刀，眼科剪刀，眼科镊子，缝衣针，棉线，注射器，台式营养器，台氏液，1×10^{-4} mol/L 组胺，1×10^{-6} mol/L 组胺，1×10^{-5} mol/L 苯海拉明，1% $BaCl_2$。

【实验步骤及观察项目】

1. 制备豚鼠回肠平滑肌标本　取豚鼠一只，用木棒猛击头部致死，迅速解剖腹腔，首先找到膨大的回盲部，然后沿着回盲部逆行寻找，与回盲部相连的即回肠，如图 4 - 7 所示，剪 5～6 cm 置于台氏液中（饱和氧状态）。将肠系膜及少量脂肪清除，用眼科剪剪成 1.5～2 cm 左右长的回肠环。肠管的对角线分别与张力换能器和肌槽内的钩子上相连，悬挂回肠环时，不能过度牵拉回肠环，以免脱钩破坏回肠。将张力换能器信号输入 BL - 420 生物机能实验系统，调整相关参数，达到最佳状态。平滑肌槽内充有台氏液，水温保持在（38±0.5）℃，并含有饱和的氧气。平衡回肠环的正常负荷。

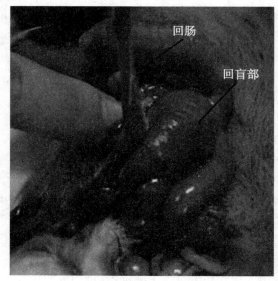

图 4 - 7　豚鼠回盲部

Fig. 4 - 7　Ileocecum of guinea pig

2. 不同剂量的组胺收缩回肠平滑肌的作用　待肠管张力稳定后，将张力调至尽量接近零点处，记录最初的台氏液体积，加入 1×10^{-6} mol/L 组胺 0.5 ml，观察回肠环张力变化情况并记录。用台氏液间断冲洗标本 3 次，加入台氏液达到原本的体积。待回肠环张力恢复稳定后，加入 1×10^{-4} mol/L 组胺 0.5 ml，观察回肠环张力变化情况并记录。

3. 苯海拉明的拮抗作用和组胺的回复作用　清洗组胺作用后的肠管，待平衡稳定后，加入 1×10^{-5} mol/L 苯海拉明 0.5 ml，记录加药后平滑肌槽中张力变化；再加入 1×10^{-6} mol/L 组胺 0.5 ml，观察张力曲线的变化；最后加入 0.5 ml 1×10^{-4} mol/L 组胺，观察并绘制张力曲线的变化。

4. $BaCl_2$ 对平滑肌的作用　加入 1% $BaCl_2$ 0.5 ml，观察张力曲线的变化。

【注意事项】

1. 制备组织标本时应小心谨慎，避免牵拉、损坏。

2. 实验中注意浴槽内温度恒定，并不断给予空气。

3. 肠管与换能器连接线不要太紧，也不能与浴管壁接触，实验中不可改变记录仪的灵敏度及标本的负荷。

4. 向浴管内加药时不要滴在线及管壁上，应将药液直接滴在液面上。

【思考题】

1. 什么是激动药与拮抗药？它们有何特点？

2. 简述组胺受体激动药以及拮抗药的作用和机制？

（韩　婷）

Experiment 16　The competitive antagonistic effect of diphenhydramine on histamine

[**Experimental objective**]　To observe the action of histamine on the intestinal smooth muscle and the competitive antagonistic effect of diphenhydramine.

[**Experimental principles**]　Histamine is an active substance widely present in tissues. Histamine can bind with histamine receptors (H_1, H_2, and H_3) on the target cells, to produce a variety of biological effects. H_1 - receptors are distributed in various kinds of smooth muscles. Guinea-pig ileum is particularly sensitive to histamine. Competitive antagonist, a drug that lacks intrinsic efficacy but retains affinity competes with the agonist for the binding site on the receptor. The characteristic pattern of such antagonism is the concentration-dependent production of a parallel shift to the right of the agonist dose-response curve with no change in the maximal asymptotic response. Diphenhydramine is a competitive antagonist of histamine; it can block the binding of histamine with the H_1 receptor, to produce anti-histamine effect.

[**Experimental object**]　guinea pig, 250 – 300 g

[**Experimental materials**]　Organ-bath, tension transducer, BL – 420 biologic experimental system, Tyrode's solution, Histamine (1×10^{-4} mol/L and 1×10^{-6} mol/L), diphenhydramine solution (1×10^{-5} mol/L), 1% $BaCl_2$

[**Experimental procedures and observational items**]

1. Preparation of guinea-pig ileum specimen　Kill the guinea pig by a knock on the head. Expose the abdominal cavity quickly and then isolate the ileum. Cut off the ileum close to the ileocecal junction (Fig. 4 – 8), and place it in a dish containing enough cold Tyrode's solution saturated with mixed oxygen. Remove the connective tissues and fat tissues around the ileum, and then cut into rings of approximately 1. 5 – 2 cm. A thread is attached to each end by inserting a needle from the inside of the gut outwards. The guinea-pig ileum is suspended in the organ-bath containing Tyrode's solution (pH 7. 4) at ($38 \pm 0. 5$)℃ and the load should be about 0. 5 g. Connect the aerator to blow the air. Turn on the recorder and record a length of base line until the base line become steady.

2. Action of 1×10^{-6} mol/L histamine　When the spontaneous rhythmicity of ileum is weak, adjust the recording trace to the baseline, add 1×10^{-6} mol/L histamine 0. 5 ml and observe and draw the contraction reaction's curve of ileum. When the contraction plateau ap-

pears, wash histamine with Tyrode's solution three times to allow the line to normalize to base level.

3. Action of 1×10^{-4} mol/L histamine   Observe the contraction reaction of ileum by adding 1×10^{-4} mol/L histamine 0.5 ml. When the contraction plateau appears, wash histamine three times to allow the line to return to base level. Observe and draw the contraction reaction's curve of ileum.

4. Competitive antagonistic effect of diphenhydramine   Add 1×10^{-5} mol/L diphenhydramine solution 0.5 ml and wait for 1 minute and observe the contraction reaction, then add 1×10^{-6} mol/L histamine 0.5 ml and observe the alteration of curve. 1 minute later, add 1×10^{-4} mol/L histamine 0.5 ml, observe and draw the alteration of curve.

5. Action of 1% $BaCl_2$ Add 1% $BaCl_2$ solution 0.5 ml and observe the alteration of curve.

[Precautions]

1. Preparation of tissue specimens should be carried out with care to protect the ileum from excess damage. Avoid excessive pulling and oppression.

2. Keep the temperature of the bath constant, and supply the air continuously.

3. The connection line between the ileum and the transducer shall not be too tight, nor in contact with the bath wall. Do not arbitrarily change the parameters of biological signal acquisition system and the sample load.

4. When adding the drugs, do not touch the cable and bath walls; it should directly drip in the liquid.

[Questions]

1. What are the characteristics agonists and antagonists and the characteristics?

2. What are the roles and mechanisms of agonists and antagonists of the histamine receptors?

（Han Ting）

实验十七　拟、抗肾上腺素药对家兔心率和血压的影响

【实验目的】　观察拟肾上腺素药物对家兔心率、血压的作用及抗肾上腺素药物对其作用的影响；分析各药对肾上腺素受体的作用。

【实验原理】　血压形成与心室射血、血管阻力和循环血量三个基本因素相关，通过神经-体液调节机制维持正常血压。拟、抗肾上腺素药物通过激动或阻断分布于心脏、血管上的肾上腺素受体，影响心肌收缩频率、血管舒缩程度从而影响心率和血压。

【实验对象】　家兔，体重 2～3 kg，雌雄均可

【实验用品】　10^{-5} mol/L 肾上腺素，10^{-4} mol/L 肾上腺素，10^{-5} mol/L 去甲肾上腺素，10^{-5} mol/L 异丙肾上腺素，1%酚妥拉明，0.1%普萘洛尔，5%枸橼酸钠，1%肝素，25%乌拉坦，生理盐水，兔解剖台，BL-420 生物机能实验系统，动脉套管，动脉夹，手术器械，丝线，头皮针，注射器，小烧杯

【实验步骤与观察项目】

1. 家兔麻醉　家兔称重后，用 25％乌拉坦按 4 ml/kg 耳缘静脉注射麻醉，仰卧固定。（注意：耳缘静脉麻醉用硅胶管头皮针，注射麻醉药后保留该头皮针，并用胶布固定，末端连接充满生理盐水的注射器，备注射药物用。）

2. 分离颈总动脉　剪去颈前部兔毛，正中切开皮肤 5～6 cm，用止血钳纵向分离软组织及颈部肌肉，暴露气管及与气管平行的血管神经鞘，在左侧颈总动脉下置细线两根，结扎其远心端，并在近心端夹上动脉夹以阻断血流。

3. 颈总动脉插管　在结扎下方的动脉上用眼科剪剪一"V"形切口，将连于压力换能器的已充满肝素生理盐水的动脉插管向心脏方向插入颈动脉内，用线扎紧固定。

4. 肝素化　耳缘静脉注入 0.5％肝素生理盐水溶液 1 ml/kg，以防止凝血。

5. 记录血压　打开动脉夹，待血压稳定后，描记一段正常曲线，并记录。

6. 给药　由耳缘静脉给药，给药顺序如下。每次给药后，迅速以 0.5 ml 生理盐水冲洗静脉管，使残余在插管内的药液进入静脉，记录血压曲线，待血压平稳后再给下一药物。

（1）观察拟肾上腺素药物的作用。

① 10^{-5} mol/L 肾上腺素 0.2 ml/kg（如无后 β 效应，改用 10^{-4} mol/L 肾上腺素 0.2 ml/kg）

② 10^{-5} mol/L 去甲肾上腺素 0.2 ml/kg

③ 10^{-5} mol/L 异丙肾上腺素 0.2 ml/kg

（2）观察应用 α-肾上腺素能受体阻断剂后对拟肾上腺素药物作用的影响。

① 1％酚妥拉明 0.5 ml/kg，用药后 2～5 min 再给下列药液

② 重复（1）中 ②

③ 重复（1）中 ①

④ 重复（1）中 ③

（3）观察应用 β-肾上腺素能受体阻断剂后对拟肾上腺素药物作用的影响。

① 0.1％普萘洛尔 0.4 ml/kg，缓慢注入用药后约 5 min 再给下列药物

② 重复（1）中 ③

③ 重复（1）中 ②

④ 重复（1）中 ①

实验数据填入表 4 - 10 和表 4 - 11。

表 4 - 10　肾上腺素、去甲肾上腺素、异丙肾上腺素对家兔血压的影响
Tab. 4 - 10　Effect of AD, NA and ISO on blood pressure of rabbits

药物 Drug	给药剂量 Dosage	受体阻断前 Before blocking	酚妥拉明给药后 After Phen	普纳洛尔给药后 After Prop
肾上腺素 AD				
去甲肾上腺素 NA				
异丙肾上腺素 ISO				

表 4 - 11 　AD、NA、ISO 对家兔心率的影响

Tab. 4 - 11 　Effect of AD, NA and ISO on heart rate of rabbits

药物 Drug	给药剂量 Dosage	受体阻断前 Before blocking	酚妥拉明给药后 After Phen	普纳洛尔给药后 After Prop
肾上腺素 AD				
去甲肾上腺素 NA				
异丙肾上腺素 ISO				

【注意事项】

1. 麻醉时，耳缘静脉注射要从其远端开始，注射速度缓慢并密切观察动物呼吸、角膜反射情况。

2. 分离血管动作要轻，不要过分拉扯，以防弄破血管。

3. 在切开动脉前必须用动脉夹夹住动脉。

4. 待前面一个药物作用基本消失后，再注射下一个药物。每次给药做好标记。

5. AD、NA、ISO 注射速度要快；酚妥拉明，普萘洛尔注入时应缓慢，以免血压急剧下降造成动物死亡；给阻断剂后，应抓紧时机注入激动剂。

【思考题】

1. 讨论各药对血压和心率的作用特点。

2. 从受体理论分析并解释各药对血压和心率的影响。

（韩淑英）

Experiment 17　Effect of adrenomimetic drugs and antiadrenergic drugs on heart rate and blood pressure in rabbits

[**Experimental objectives**]　To observe the effect of adrenomimetic drugs and the effect of antiadrenergic drugs on electrocardiogram and blood pressure in rabbits; to analyze the effect of the drugs on the adrenergic receptor.

[**Experimental principles**]　Formation of blood pressure is associated with three basic factors ventricular ejection, vascular resistance and circulating blood volume. Normal blood pressure is maintained by neural-humoral regulation mechanism. Adrenomimetic drugs and antiadrenergic drugs affect heart rate and blood pressure by stimulating or blocking adrenergic receptor of the heart and blood vessels.

[**Experimental object**]　rabbit (2 - 3 kg)

[**Experimental materials**]　10^{-5} mol/L adrenaline (AD), 10^{-4} mol/L adrenaline, 10^{-5} mol/L noradrenaline (NA), 10^{-5} mol/L isoprenaline (ISO), 1% phentolamine (Phen), 0.1% propranolol (Prop), 5% sodium citrate, 1% heparin, 25% urethane, normal saline, rabbit dissecting table, BL - 420 system, arterial cannula, arterial clamp, surgical instruments, silk suture, scalp venous needle, injection syringe, beaker

[Experimental procedures and observation items]

1. Anesthesia and fixation The rabbit is weighed and injected with 25% ethylcarbamate (4 ml/kg) via the marginal ear vein through a scalp venous indwelling needle.

2. Separation of common carotid artery After 5 – 6 cm skin incision is cut in the center of the neck, the soft tissues and muscles are separated with hemostatic forceps to expose the left carotid artery. Then two threads are put down under the carotid artery, the distal end is ligated and the proximal end is clamped to block blood flow.

3. Carotid artery cannulation Arterial cannula is inserted into the common carotid artery and fixed with silk suture.

4. Heparinization in body Heparin (1 ml/kg) is injected through the marginal ear vein to avoid coagulation.

5. Blood pressure record BL – 420 system is started to record normal blood pressure after the observed blood pressure becomes stable.

6. Administration The sequence of drugs given is as below. After each administration, flush venous duct with 0.5 ml saline quickly to flush the residual liquid in the cannula out into the vein and then record blood pressure curve. The next drug is given after blood pressure has been stabilized.

(1) To observe the effect of adrenomimetic drugs.

① 10^{-5} mol/L AD, 0.2 ml/kg (if no post-β effect appears, 10^{-4} mol/L AD given, 0.2 ml/kg)

② 10^{-5} mol/L NA, 0.2 ml/kg

③ 10^{-5} mol/L ISO, 0.2 ml/kg

(2) To observe the effect of α-adrenergic receptor blocker on adrenomimetic drugs.

① 1% Phen 0.5 ml/kg (give the following drugs after 2 – 5 min)

② 10^{-5} mol/L NA, 0.2 ml/kg

③ 10^{-5} mol/L AD, 0.2 ml/kg

④ 10^{-5} mol/L ISO, 0.2 ml/kg

(3) To observe the effect of β-adrenergic receptor blocker on adrenomimetic drugs.

① 1% Prop 0.4 ml/kg (give the following drugs after 5 min)

② 10^{-5} mol/L NA, 0.2 ml/kg

③ 10^{-4} mol/L AD, 0.2 ml/kg

④ 10^{-5} mol/L ISO, 0.2 ml/kg

The experimental results should be filled in Tab. 4 – 10 and Tab. 4 – 11.

[Precautions]

1. During anesthesia, the marginal ear vein injection should begin from the far end with slow injection speed and breathing and corneal reflection closely.

2. Blood vessels should be separated softly in case excessive pulling breaks the vessels.

3. The artery must be clamped by an artery clamp before it is cut.

4. The next drug should not be given until the effect of the last drug disappears completely.

5. AD, NA and ISO should be injected rapidly, Phen and Prop should be injected slowly in order to avoid death of the animal due to a sharp decline in the blood pressure. The agonist should be injected immediately after antagonist injection.

[**Questions**]

1. Discuss functional characteristics of adrenomimetic drugs and antiadrenergic drugs on blood pressure and heart rate.

2. Analyze and explain the effect of the drugs on blood pressure and heart rate from the receptor theory perspective.

(Bai Jing)

实验十八　高钾血症对心脏的影响及抢救

【实验目的】　掌握家兔高钾血症模型的复制方法，设计抢救治疗方案；观察家兔心脏及心电图的变化，掌握血钾升高对心脏的毒性作用。

【实验原理】　耳缘静脉注射氯化钾溶液使家兔钾摄入过多，制作高钾血症动物模型。血钾浓度升高可影响心肌的兴奋性、传导性、自律性和收缩性，这些生理特性的变化可以引起心电图的相应改变以及心脏搏动状态的变化。通过开胸暴露心脏和描记心电图，观察血钾升高对心脏的毒性作用。碳酸氢钠可拮抗此毒性作用，当出现严重心律失常时用碳酸氢钠进行解救并观察其疗效。

【实验对象】　家兔

【实验用品】　兔台，BL-420生物机能实验系统，手术器械，注射器（5 ml、10 ml），头皮针，25%氨基甲酸乙酯（乌拉坦）溶液，（2%、5%、10%）氯化钾溶液，生理盐水，4%碳酸氢钠溶液，手术线，纱布

【实验步骤】

1. 麻醉、固定　取兔一只并称重，25%乌拉坦（4 ml/kg）耳缘静脉缓慢注射麻醉动物，将其仰卧位固定于兔台，左胸部剪毛。

2. 开胸手术　胸锁关节水平沿胸壁正中线向下做皮肤切口6～7 cm，用手术刀剥离左侧胸壁肌肉暴露肋骨并计数，出血时以湿生理盐水纱布按压止血。确认开胸暴露心脏的最佳位置，一般在胸骨左缘与第4肋下缘的交界点。从此处向上剪断第4和第3肋骨，打开胸腔，即可观察到搏动的心脏。用手指轻触心脏，感受心脏搏动的节律和力度，观察心脏的大小、颜色等一般状态。

3. 心电图观察　将与BL-420相连的针形电极插入家兔四肢皮下，导联线按右前肢—红，左前肢—黄，右后肢—黑的对应关系连接。观察家兔正常心电图，记录1～2个心动周期的心电波形。

4. 制作动物模型　用注射器抽取2%氯化钾溶液（1 ml/kg）排空气泡待用，将充有生理盐水的头皮针刺入耳缘静脉，见到回血后推注少量液体，固定针头。接注射器并缓慢推注2%氯化钾溶液，每间隔3 min给药1次，反复3次。然后依次换用5%和10%氯化钾溶液，方法和用量同上。在推注氯化钾过程中要密切观察和记录心电图及心脏活动的变化特征，一旦出现室颤及时停止给药。

5. 抢救　待心脏出现心室扑动或颤动后立即停止注射氯化钾溶液，迅速由耳缘静脉注入已备好的抢救药物 4% 碳酸氢钠溶液（5 ml/kg），同时辅以心脏按压促进心脏复跳。

6. 致死　对于抢救成功的动物，注入致死量的 10% 氯化钾溶液（8 ml/kg），观察心肌纤颤及心脏停搏时的状态。

【观察项目】

1. 高血钾前后家兔心脏形态及搏动的状态。

2. 高血钾前后家兔心电图的特征。

【注意事项】

1. 开胸时注意止血，避免出现气胸，尤其是左侧气胸。

2. 室颤可能发生在 3 种浓度氯化钾溶液各 3 次的注射过程中的任意一步，应密切注意观察。一旦出现，及时停止给药。

3. 保持实验室安静和实验台的整洁，减轻心电干扰。

4. 保持家兔耳缘静脉通畅，抢救药物应在室颤发生后 10 s 内快速注入，否则救治效果不佳。

【思考题】

1. 除静脉途径摄钾过多外，临床上引起高钾血症的原因还有哪些？

2. 碳酸氢钠救治高钾血症的机制是什么？还有哪些其他救治措施？机制如何？

（赵利军　门秀丽）

Experiment 18　Effect of hyperkalemia on the heart

〔**Experimental objectives**〕　To duplicate the animal model of hyperkalemia in rabbit; to observe the effect of hyperkalemia on the heart. To understand the characteristic of ECG during hyperkalemia.

〔**Experimental principles**〕　The animal model of hyperkalemia is duplicated in rabbit via the marginal ear vein injection of KCl. Hyperkalemia can affect cardiac excitability, conductivity, autorhythmicity and contractility. These changes of myocardial physiological characteristics can cause ECG changes. The ECG to be recorded observe the toxicity of hyperkalemia on the heart. And the rabbit is then rescued with $NaHCO_3$.

〔**Experimental object**〕　rabbit

〔**Experimental materials**〕　BL - 420, surgical instruments, syringes (5 ml, 10 ml), scalp needle, 25% urethane, (2%, 5%, 10%) KCl, normal saline, 4% $NaHCO_3$

〔**Experimental procedures**〕

1. Anaesthesia and restraint　Weigh the rabbit. Induce general anaesthesia by injecting 25% urethane (4 ml/kg) via the marginal vein of the ear to make a general anaesthesia. Fix it in a dorsal position on the operating table.

2. Record of ECG　Insert needle electrodes under the skin of the animal limbs: right front limb-red, left front limb-yellow, right rear limb-black.

3. Duplication of animal model　Inject 1ml /kg of 2% KCl slowly through the ear vein

for 3 times, with a break of 3 min between each injection. And then inject successively with 5% and 10% KCl with the same dosage, until ventricular fibrillation appears. Record the ECG changes.

4. Rescue Rescue with 4% NaHCO₃ (5 ml/kg), and perform closed cardiac massage.

[**Observations**] Characteristic of ECG

[**Precautions**]

1. KCl should be injected slowly. Ventricular fibrillation may occur anytime during KCl injection. Once it occurs, stop injection immediately and rescue.

2. Avoid disturbance of surrounding magnetic fields of surrounding while making recording ECG.

[**Questions**]

1. What changes of ECG have you already observed as a result of KCl injection? And why do they appear?

2. How do you rescue your rabbit? And what is the theoretical basis?

(Wu Jing Men Xiuli)

实验十九　缺氧及抢救

一、家兔乏氧性缺氧

【实验目的】　掌握乏氧性缺氧动物模型的复制方法；观察缺氧过程中机体的代偿及失代偿变化，并分析其可能机制。

【实验原理】　利用缺氧装置使家兔吸入的气体呈氧分压逐渐降低的状态，从而使动脉血氧分压降低，制作乏氧性缺氧动物模型。缺氧对机体各个系统均有一定的影响，轻度或慢性缺氧时，机体还可出现适应代偿性变化。本实验以动物的血压、呼吸运动及皮肤黏膜颜色的变化为主要观察指标，验证乏氧性缺氧对机体的影响。

【实验对象】　家兔

【实验用品】　兔台，BL-420 生物机能实验系统，25%氨基甲酸乙酯（乌拉坦）溶液，肝素，手术器械，缺氧瓶（内装钠石灰），乳胶管（约 15 cm 长），动脉插管，气管插管，动脉夹，手术线，纱布

【实验步骤】

1. 麻醉、固定　取兔一只并称重，25%乌拉坦（4 ml/kg）耳缘静脉缓慢注射麻醉动物，将其仰卧位固定于兔台，颈部剪毛。

2. 颈部手术　颈正中线剪开皮肤 6～7 cm，钝性分离颈部肌肉，暴露气管及双侧颈总动脉，分离气管并做气管插管，注意气管插管处结扎要紧密，以防漏气。分离双侧颈总动脉并穿线备用（一侧动脉穿单线，另一侧动脉穿双线）。耳缘静脉注入肝素 1 ml/kg（1000 U/kg）。选择穿双线的动脉，结扎其远心端，动脉夹夹闭其近心端阻断血流。在靠近远心端结扎处用眼科剪剪一小"V"字形切口，将充好肝素盐水的动脉插管向心方向插入动脉并固定好动脉插

管。打开与 BL‑420 生物机能实验系统连接的三通装置，观察血压搏动曲线。

3. 观察并记录家兔正常一般状态　记录动物的血压（平均值）和心率，肉眼观察动物呼吸运动的节律、频率及胸廓运动的幅度及皮肤黏膜的颜色。用动脉夹夹闭对侧颈总动脉10～15 s，观察血压的变化，即夹闭反射试验（第 1 次）。

4. 缺氧　乳胶管接"Y"形气管插管的一侧并用止血钳夹闭，将缺氧瓶与气管插管另一侧相连，如图 4‑8 所示。记录开始缺氧的时间，并密切观察上述指标的变化。当血压降到动物正常血压的 1/2 时，进行第 2 次夹闭反射试验，方法同上，观察血压的变化。

5. 抢救　当血压下降到正常血压的 1/3 左右或低于 30 mmHg 时，停止缺氧，进行抢救。

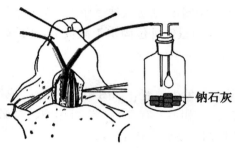

图 4‑8　缺氧瓶原理图
Fig. 4‑8　Schematics of hypoxia bottle

【观察项目】
缺氧前后家兔血压，心率，呼吸运动（频率、节律和幅度）及皮肤黏膜颜色的变化。

【注意事项】
1. 严格遵守动脉插管的注意事项，避免血液意外喷溅。
2. 注意检查气管插管三个接口处的密闭性，防止漏气。
3. 实验结束撤除动脉插管前，先将颈总动脉结扎再拔动脉插管。

【思考题】
1. 家兔缺氧后其血压和呼吸运动变化如何？分析其病理生理学机制。
2. 两次夹闭反射试验的结果及机制如何？本实验中设置此环节的意义何在？

二、小白鼠缺氧

【实验目的】　掌握小白鼠乏氧性缺氧与血液性缺氧模型的复制方法；观察并比较这两种类型缺氧对机体的影响，并分析其机制。

【实验原理】　将小白鼠放入盛有钠石灰的密闭缺氧瓶中，以模拟大气中氧分压降低，制作乏氧性缺氧动物模型。通过提高小白鼠吸入气中 CO 浓度，使其体内的血红蛋白与 CO 结合形成碳氧血红蛋白而失去携带氧气的能力，导致血液性缺氧。两种类型缺氧的发生机制不同，机体的表现也不同。

【实验对象】　小白鼠 3 只（1 号：乏氧性缺氧小白鼠；2 号：血液性缺氧小白鼠；3 号：正常小白鼠）

【实验用品】 小白鼠缺氧瓶2个，一氧化碳发生装置，钠石灰，甲酸，硫酸，5%氢氧化钠，酒精灯，10 ml注射器，手术器械，鼠板3个，橡皮筋

【实验步骤】

1. 乏氧性缺氧

（1）缺氧：随机取小白鼠一只，编为1号并标记，将其放入盛有钠石灰的缺氧瓶中，塞紧瓶塞。记录开始缺氧的时间，观察其一般状态、呼吸频率和深度、口唇黏膜和尾尖部颜色及其变化。

（2）抢救：当小白鼠出现明显的呼吸抑制时，将其从缺氧瓶中取出，轻轻挤压胸壁进行抢救。

（3）致死：若抢救成功再次将小白鼠置入缺氧瓶直至死亡。

（4）解剖观察：将死亡的小白鼠仰卧位固定于鼠板上，沿胸、腹正中线打开胸、腹腔，观察血液及内脏的颜色。

2. 血液性缺氧

（1）制取CO：连接一氧化碳发生装置，如图4-9所示，取甲酸3 ml加入试管内，再加入浓硫酸2~3 ml，塞紧试管。如不见有气泡产生可用酒精灯微微加热，但不可过热至液体沸腾。将产生的CO收集于密闭的球囊中备用。

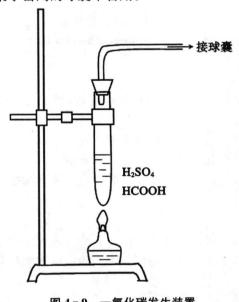

图 4 - 9　一氧化碳发生装置

Fig. 4 - 9　CO generating device

（2）缺氧：随机取小白鼠一只，编为2号并标记，将其放入广口瓶中，塞紧瓶塞。用注射器取CO 5~8 ml经注射器针头注入瓶内。随时注意观察上述指标的变化。

（3）抢救：当小白鼠严重缺氧出现抽搐时，立即将其取出置于通风处，观察动物恢复的情况。

（4）致死：若抢救成功，再次将小白鼠置入缺氧瓶，注入CO 5~8 ml。此次不抢救直至小白鼠死亡。

（5）解剖观察：解剖小白鼠观察血液及内脏的颜色。

3. 正常小鼠

（1）正常状态的观察：取小白鼠一只，编为 3 号并标记，观察其一般状态、呼吸频率和深度、口唇黏膜和尾尖部颜色等一般状态。

（2）致死并解剖：以颈椎脱臼法处死小白鼠，解剖并观察血液及内脏的颜色。

【观察项目】

1. 缺氧前后小白鼠呼吸频率和幅度的变化。

2. 正常与缺氧小白鼠不同部位颜色的观察与比较（表 4 - 12）。

3. 缺氧小白鼠的耐受缺氧时间。

表 4 - 12　小白鼠不同部位的颜色变化

Tab. 4 - 12　Color changes in different position of mice with different types of hypoxia

鼠号 Number	血液 Blood	唇 Lip	耳 Ear	四肢 Limb	尾 Tail	肝 Liver	心脏 Heart
1							
2							
3							

【注意事项】

1. 缺氧瓶瓶口一定要密闭。

2. 注入 CO 时切忌过多过快，避免动物迅速死亡而影响血液颜色的变化和观察。

3. CO 为有毒气体，应在特定的通风环境中进行制备，现用现制。

【思考题】

1. 机体皮肤黏膜颜色在这两种类型缺氧中有何特征性表现？分析其病理生理学机制。

2. 按发病机制，缺氧可分为哪几种类型？本实验中动物的缺氧类型是什么？

（赵利军　门秀丽）

Experiment 19　Hypoxia

Part 1　Hypotonic hypoxia in rabbits

[**Experimental objectives**]　To duplicate the animal model of hypotonic hypoxia in rabbit; to observe the changes of respiratory system, circulatory system, color of skin and mucosa.

[**Experimental principles**]　Hypoxia chambers are used to duplicated the animal model of hypotonic hypoxia in rabbit by decreasing PO_2 of inspired air with hypoxia bottle. The changes of the respiratory system, circulatory system, color of skin and mucosa are observed to verify the impact of hypotonic hypoxia on the body.

[**Experimental object**]　rabbit

[**Experimental materials**]　BL - 420, 25% urethane, heparin solution, surgical instruments, hypoxia bottle, rubber tube (about 15 cm long), artery cannula, tracheal cannula, artery clamp, surgical thread, gauze

[**Experimental procedures**]

1. Preoperative preparation   Weigh the rabbit. Anaesthetize it with 25% urethane (4 ml/kg) via the marginal vein of the ear for induction of general anaesthesia. Fix it in a dorsal position on the operating table.

2. Neck surgery   Shear the hair of the neck, and cut the skin along the midline for 6 – 7 cm. Separate the trachea, and perform tracheal intubation. Separate one side carotid artery. Inject heparin (1 ml/kg) via the ear vein. Then conduct carotid artery intubation with the three – way pipe connected to BL – 420 for recording arterial blood pressure.

3. Observation and record   Take notes of normal blood pressure (BP), heart rate (HR), respiratory rate (RR) and amplitude, color of skin and mucosa. Perform the depressor reflex for the first time by clamping contralateral carotid artery for 10 – 15 s, and observe changes of BP.

4. Hypotonic hypoxia   Close one end of the tracheal cannula with a rubber tube. Connect the other end of the cannula with the hypoxia chamber. Now, the animal should be under hypotonic hypoxia condition. Observe the changes of indexes every 3min. Perform the depressor reflex for the second time when BP drops to 1/2 of normal value.

5. Rescue   Remove the hypoxia chamber and rescue the rabbit when BP drops to 1/3 of normal BP or less than 30 mmHg.

[**Observations**]

Blood pressure (BP), heart rate (HR), respiratory rate (RR) and amplitude, color of skin and mucosa.

[**Precautions**]

1. Prevent leakage of artery cannula and tracheal cannula.

2. Remember to ligate the carotid artery before withdrawing artery cannula.

[**Questions**]

1. What are the different changes at different stages of hypotonic hypoxia? And what is the pathogenesis?

2. How do you explain the different results and their corresponding mechanisms for the differences in observed depressor reflexes? What's the significance of the design for this experiment?

Part 2   Hypotonic hypoxia and hemic hypoxia in mice

[**Experimental objectives**]   To duplicate the animal model of hypotonic hypoxia and hemic hypoxia in mouse; to observe the appearance during hypoxia and compare the differences between hypoxic hypoxia and hemic hypoxia.

[**Experimental principles**]   The mouse is placed in a sealed hypoxia bottle to duplicate

90

the animal model of hypotonic hypoxia. The concentration of CO is increased in the air inhaled by the mouse so the body's hemoglobin forms carboxyhemoglobin with CO and loses the ability to carry oxygen, resulting in hemic hypoxia. The mice show different body reactions to these two types of hypoxia with different mechanisms.

[**Experimental object**]　mouse

[**Experimental materials**]　Wide-neck bottles, devices of acute operation, sodica calx (sodium hydrate + calcium oxide), 10 ml syringe, HCOOH, H_2SO_4

[**Experimental procedures**]

1. Hypotonic hypoxia

(1) Hypoxia　Take a mouse. Put it into the wide-neck bottle which has some sodica calx in the bottom. Then stopper the bottle tightly without any ventilation, make record of time. Observe the appearance of the mouse, the movement and the color change of its lips, ears and limbs etc. Count the respiratory rate every 5 min.

(2) Rescue　Remove the stopper and take out the mouse when the mouse showed severe respiratory depression. Gently compress the chest to rescue.

(3) Execution　Pat the rescued mouse back into the hypoxia bottle until it dies.

(4) Observation　Open the abdominal cavity and the thoracic cavity to examine the color of internal organs, such as the liver and the heart of the mouse.

2. Hemic hypoxia (Isotonic hypoxia): CO poisoning

(1) Preparation of CO　Use the equipment shown in Fig. 4 - 9.

(2) Hypoxia　Get another mouse, and put it into another wide-neck bottle. Stopper the bottle tightly. Inject 5 - 8 ml CO into the bottle through the rubber tube. Observe the appearance of the mouse carefully.

(3) Rescue　Take off the stopper and put the mouse in a ventilated place when the mouse shows severe respiratory depression.

(4) Execution　Put the rescue mouse back into the bottle with 5 - 8 ml CO injection until it dies.

(5) Observation　Examine the color of the internal organs of the mouse.

3. Normal mouse as the control:

(1) Observation of the normal state　Take a normal mouse as the control and observe the appearance, respiratory rate and depth, color of lips, ears and limbs and so on.

(2) Execution　Sacrifice the normal mouse by cervical dislocation, dissect it to examine the color of the internal organs and blood.

[**Observations**]

1. Respiratory rate

2. Color difference

3. Tolerance time of the hypoxia mice

[**Precautions**]

1. Stopper the wide-neck bottle tightly.

2. Avoid injecting CO too much and too fast, or the animal will die immediately without

significant color change

3. Avoid CO poisoning due to breathing in the CO gas.

[**Questions**]

1. Why do the three mice show different colors in their bodies? Analyze pathogenesis of these two types of hypoxia.

2. What are the types of hypoxia according to the pathogenesis? What types are involved in this experiment?

（Wu Jing　Men Xiuli）

实验二十　血氨升高在肝性脑病发生中的作用

【实验目的】　掌握肝性脑病动物模型的复制方法；观察血氨升高在肝性脑病发生中的作用，并分析其可能机制。

【实验原理】　肝性脑病是继发于严重肝功能障碍的神经精神综合征。本实验通过结扎家兔大部分肝叶而阻断血供，造成肝解毒功能急剧障碍；再经十二指肠注入复方氯化铵溶液，导致肠道氨的生成增多并吸收入血。由于氨的清除不足与摄入过多同时存在，血氨迅速升高引起氨中毒。氨可通过血脑屏障干扰脑细胞的功能和代谢，从而使家兔逐渐出现肝性脑病的典型表现。

【实验对象】　家兔

【实验用品】　兔台，1％普鲁卡因溶液，手术器械，粗棉线，三通塑料插管，氯化铵，葡萄糖，碳酸氢钠，注射器（5 ml、10 ml），手术线，纱布

【实验步骤】

1. 麻醉固定　取兔一只并称重，将其仰卧位固定于兔台，上腹部剪毛，沿腹正中线在腹壁上用1％普鲁卡因做局部多点浸润麻醉。

2. 开腹并结扎肝叶　自胸骨剑突向下，沿腹正中线作一6～8 cm皮肤切口。沿腹白线打开腹腔，观察正常腹腔的一般状态。在右上腹暴露出肝，术者左手示指和中指在肝镰状韧带两侧将肝轻轻下压，右手持眼科剪剪断肝与膈肌之间的镰状韧带。然后再将肝向上翻，剪断肝与胃之间的肝胃韧带。辨明肝各叶，用粗棉线环绕结扎肝右中叶、左中叶、左外叶，保留右外叶和尾状叶。

3. 十二指肠插管　沿胃幽门向右后下方向找出十二指肠并穿线，在十二指肠上剪一小口，将带有三通的塑料插管向尾端方向插入十二指肠并固定。用两把止血钳夹闭腹壁皮肤切缘关闭腹腔，将三通管尾端留置在外。

4. 观察正常状态　观察家兔的呼吸、角膜反射、瞳孔大小、肌张力及对刺激的反应。

5. 给药并观察　自十二指肠插管注入复方氯化铵溶液每次5 ml/kg，每隔3 min给药1次。注意观察动物有无呼吸加速、反应性增强、肌肉痉挛、抽搐等，直至动物出现全身性抽搐、角弓反张时停止给药。

6. 计算　计算复方氯化铵总用量（ml）。

【观察项目】

1. 肝性脑病前后动物呼吸、角膜反射、瞳孔大小、肌张力等指标的观察。

2. 肝性脑病动物扑翼样震颤、角弓反张、抽搐等现象。

3. 氯化铵总用量。

【注意事项】

1. 本实验全程中动物均为清醒状态，各项操作动作宜轻柔且保持实验室环境安静。

2. 剪镰状韧带时勿损伤膈肌和血管，结扎线应结扎于肝叶根部血管处，避免直接结扎肝。

3. 十二指肠插管应插向小肠方向，而不是胃、食管方向。

【思考题】

1. 本实验麻醉动物时为什么不能应用乌拉坦溶液？

2. 本实验中血氨升高的具体机制是什么？

3. 血氨升高对脑有何毒性作用？

（赵利军　门秀丽）

Experiment 20　Hepatic encephalopathy

［**Experimental objectives**］　To duplicate the animal model of hepatic encephalopathy in rabbit；to observe the effect of ammonia in pathogenesis of hepatic encephalopathy.

［**Experimental principles**］　Hepatic encephalopathy is a neuropsychiatric syndrome secondary to severe liver dysfunction. Most of the lobes of the liver in rabbits are ligated to cause acute disorder of hepatic detoxification function. Then the compound NH_4Cl solution is injected via duodenal intubation，leading to increased production of ammonia in the intestinal tract. The rabbit appears typical manifestation of hepatic encephalopathy gradually with elevated blood ammonia.

［**Experimental object**］　rabbit

［**Experimental materials**］　1% procaine solution，surgical instruments，thick thread，three-way plastic cannula，compound NH_4Cl solution，syringes（5 ml，10 ml），surgical thread，gauze

［**Experimental procedures**］

1. Preoperative preparation　Weigh the rabbit and fix it in a dorsal position on the operating table. Shear the hair of the abdomen. Induce a local anesthesia by injecting 1% procaine along the midline of the abdomen.

2. Laparotomy and ligation of the hepatic lobes　Cut the skin along the midline of the abdomen. Open the abdominal cavity. Press the liver downward softly，and observe the five lobes of liver. Cut off the ligament which is located between the liver and diaphragm. Tie the roots of liver lobes with thick thread to stop blood flow into liver. Then the hepatic infarction will occur infarct soon.

3. Duodenal intubation　Toward the intestine，insert a three-way plastic cannula into duodenum and fix it.

4. Observations　Observe the breathing，corneal reflex，pupil size，muscle tension and

response to stimuli.

5. Administration and observation Inject compound NH_4Cl solution to the duodenum at the dosage of 5 ml/kg each time, with a break of 3 min between each injection. Observe the breathing, corneal reflex, pupil size, muscle tension, flapping tremor and convulsions until opisthotonos appear.

6. Calculation Count the total volume of the drug that has been used.

[Observational items]

Breathing, corneal reflex, pupil size, muscle tension, flapping tremor, opisthotonos, convulsions, total amount of NH_4Cl solution.

[Precautions]

1. Do not injure the diaphragm and vessels when cutting off the ligament between the liver and the diaphragm. Ligature should be tied at the lobe roots, to avoid hepatic lobes injury.

2. The three-way plastic cannula should be inserted into the duodenum toward the direction of the intestines but not in the direction of the stomach.

[Questions]

1. Why do we use procaine instead of urethane solution as the anesthetic in this experiment?

2. Try to explain the ammonia's role in pathogenesis of hepatic encephalopathy.

(Wu Jing Men Xiuli)

实验二十一 急性肺水肿

【实验目的】 掌握家兔实验性肺水肿动物模型的复制方法；观察肺水肿的表现，分析肺水肿形成的有关机制。

【实验原理】 组织液的生成大于回流是引起血管内外液体交换失平衡并导致水肿的重要机制。本实验通过颈外静脉快速、大量输注生理盐水，升高毛细血管流体静压、降低血浆胶体渗透压。再加入肾上腺素使血液由体循环急速转入肺循环，导致肺组织液的生成大于回流，引发肺水肿。通过观察动物的呼吸运动、呼吸音及肺大体形态的变化，探讨肺水肿对机体的影响。

【实验对象】 家兔

【实验用品】 兔台，25%氨基甲酸乙酯（乌拉坦）溶液，手术器械，气管插管，注射器（5 ml、10 ml），头皮针，静脉输液装置，静脉导管，听诊器，滤纸，手术线，纱布，托盘天平，生理盐水，肾上腺素

【实验步骤】

1. 麻醉固定 取兔一只并称重，25%乌拉坦（4 ml/kg）耳缘静脉缓慢注射麻醉动物，将其仰卧位固定于兔台，颈部剪毛。

2. 颈部手术 颈正中线剪开皮肤6～7 cm，钝性分离颈部肌肉，暴露气管及一侧颈外静脉，分离气管并做气管插管。把输液导管与静脉输液装置相连接，注意排除管道内气体。分

离一侧颈外静脉并穿双线，先用动脉夹夹闭其近心端阻断回心血流使静脉充盈，然后用手术线结扎其远心端，在靠远心端结扎处用眼科剪剪一小切口，将静脉导管插入约 1～2 cm 后固定，松开动脉夹，打开静脉输液装置试行滴注，通畅后暂停输液。

3. 正常状态的观察　观察并记录正常的呼吸运动（呼吸频率和胸廓运动的幅度），用听诊器听诊双肺的呼吸音。

4. 输液　取 37 ℃生理盐水，总量按照 80 ml/kg 计，加入输液瓶中。输液速度调至 150～180 滴/min。当液体输入总量的 2/3 时，向输液瓶中加入肾上腺素溶液 0.5 mg/kg 体重并轻轻摇动输液瓶使其混匀。待液体输完时再加入少量生理盐水，缓慢滴注维持通道畅通，以利必要时再次用药。

5. 动物模型的观察　观察并记录呼吸频率和胸廓运动幅度的变化，并注意用听诊器听诊肺部有无湿啰音出现。观察气管插管口是否有粉红色泡沫样液体流出。如上述现象不明显可重复使用肾上腺素，用法及剂量同上，直至出现明显的肺水肿表现。

6. 开胸取肺　当听到湿性啰音或观察到气管插管口有粉红色泡沫液流出时，用止血钳于气管插管的下端夹住气管并上提，手术剪打开胸腔，轻轻将肺和心脏一同取出，然后小心将心脏及其血管剪除。用滤纸吸干肺表面的血迹后称取肺重，计算肺系数。肺系数＝肺重量（g）/体质量（kg）（兔正常肺系数约为 4～5）。

7. 病理形态学观察　肉眼观察肺体积、颜色、质地、被膜、淤血、出血等大体改变。切开肺，观察切面有无泡沫样液体流出。

【观察项目】
1. 肺水肿发生前后动物呼吸运动及呼吸音的变化。
2. 离体肺大体表面及切面形态观察。
3. 肺系数。

【注意事项】
1. 颈外静脉分离尽可能长且干净，以确保静脉插管一次成功。
2. 静脉输液过程中，注意排空气泡。
3. 解剖取出肺时，勿挤压肺或损伤肺表面，以防止水肿液流出，影响肺系数值。

【思考题】
1. 本实验动物模型制作的原理如何？
2. 粉红色泡沫样液体出现的具体机制如何？

（赵利军　门秀丽）

Experiment 21　Experimental pulmonary edema

[**Experimental objectives**]　To duplicate the animal model of pulmonary edema in rabbit; to observe the manifestations of the animal.

[**Experimental principles**]　Pulmonary edema is induced by disturbance of transcapillary fluid exchange in the lung. In this experiment, the quick and vast normal saline infusion via the marginal ear vein may increase capillary hydrostatic pressure, and decrease plasma colloid osmotic pressure. In addition, epinephrine can switch blood from the systemic circulation into the pulmonary circulation. When combined together, these factors lead to more fluid being filtered than can be reabsorbed, causing pulmonary edema.

[**Experimental object**]　rabbit

[**Experimental materials**]　25% urethane, surgical instruments, tracheal cannula, syringes (5 ml, 10 ml), scalp needle, intravenous infusion device, intravenous catheters, stethoscope, filter paper, surgical thread, gauze, pallet scales, 0.9% normal saline, epinephrine

[**Experimental procedures**]

1. Preoperative preparation　Weigh the rabbit. Anaesthetize it with 25% urethane (4 ml/kg) via the marginal vein of the ear to induce a general anaesthesia. Fix it in a dorsal position on the operating table.

2. Neck surgery　Shear the hair of the neck, cut the skin along the midline. Separate the trachea, and perform tracheal intubation. Connect the intravenous cannula with the infusion device. Separate an external jugular vein and conduct venous cannulation. Give normal saline through intravenous infusion at 5 – 10 drops / min.

3. Observation on the normal state　Observe and record the normal breathing (respiratory rate, amplitude and sounds).

4. Intravenous　infusion infuse 80 ml/kg of saline at 150 – 180 drops / min. When 2/3 of liquid has been infused, add 0.45 mg/kg of epinephrine in the saline.

5. Observation on the animal model　Record the changes of the respiratory rate and amplitude, and check for the appearance of rales and pink foamy liquid in the tracheal cannula.

6. Thoracotomy　Appearance of rales and pink foamy liquid in the tracheal cannula indicates the formation of pulmonary edema. Clamp the trachea with a hemostatic clamp. Open the chest. Remove the lung, and weigh them. Calculate the lung coefficient. Lung weight (g) /body weight (kg), the normal value is about 4 – 5.

7. Pathological morphology　Observe the status of lung volume, color, texture, coatings, congestion and hemorrhage. Cut the lung to observe whether there is an outflow of foamy liquid.

[**Observations**]　Breathing, breath sounds, rales, general and sectional lung morphology, lung coefficient

[**Precautions**]

1. Separate a sufficiently long enough length of external jugular vein and clean other tissues away from it, in order to ensure a successful venous intubation.

2. Avoid bubbles during the intravenous infusion.

3. Do not injure the lungs when removing them, or the edema fluid outflow may affect lung coefficient.

[**Questions**]

1. What's the mechanism of experimental pulmonary edema?

2. Why does pink foamy liquid appear?

(Wu Jing　Men Xiuli)

实验二十二　失血性休克及抢救

【实验目的】　掌握失血性休克动物模型的复制方法；观察失血性休克时动物的代偿及失代偿表现，并分析其发生机制。

【实验原理】　失血性休克的发生取决于机体的失血量和失血速度。本实验通过股动脉快速放血超过总血量 30%，造成有效循环血量锐减。同时体内应激反应发生，交感-肾上腺髓质系统兴奋，儿茶酚胺释放入血增多，外周血管收缩，组织器官微循环灌流量急剧减少，重要器官及细胞功能严重障碍，引发休克。观察机体的变化，探讨失血性休克对机体的影响。

【实验对象】　家兔

【实验用品】　兔台，BL-420 生物机能实验系统，25% 乌拉坦溶液，手术器械，肝素，注射器（5 ml，50 ml），动脉导管（2 个），静脉导管，三通（3 个），气管插管，动脉夹，手术线，纱布

【实验步骤】

1. 麻醉固定　取兔一只并称重，25% 乌拉坦（4 ml/kg）耳缘静脉缓慢注射麻醉动物，将其仰卧位固定于兔台，颈部及一侧腹股沟部剪毛。

2. 颈部手术　颈正中线剪开皮肤 6～7 cm，钝性分离颈部肌肉暴露气管，分离气管并做气管插管。分离一侧颈总动脉及另一侧颈外静脉分别穿线备用。耳缘静脉注入肝素 1 ml/kg（1000 U/kg）。结扎颈总动脉远心端，动脉夹夹闭其近心端。在阻断血流段靠近头端处用眼科剪剪一小切口，将动脉插管插入并固定。打开三通，观察有无血压波动曲线。对侧做颈静脉插管，缓慢推注少量生理盐水以保持管道通畅。

3. 正常状态的观察　观察并记录家兔正常状态下的一般情况、皮肤黏膜颜色、心率、血压、呼吸。

4. 失血　在一侧腹股沟区沿股动脉走行方向做 4 cm 长的皮肤切口，分离股动脉并穿线，插入动脉导管，并与经肝素冲洗过的 50 ml 无菌注射器相连。在 BL-420 血压监测下，用注射器抽取动脉血。当血压下降至正常水平 1/3 时，关闭三通停止放血。观察家兔有无代偿性血压升高，观察休克过程中上述其他指标的变化。

5. 抢救　当血压失代偿性下降时，将注射器中的血液经颈静脉插管推注进体内，观察家兔血压及各项指标的变化。

【观察项目】　失血性休克发生前后动物一般情况、皮肤黏膜颜色、心率、血压、呼吸的变化。

【注意事项】

1. 麻醉深浅要适度。麻醉过浅，动物可因剧烈疼痛致神经源性休克；麻醉过深则抑制呼吸。

2. 手术过程中要尽量避免意外出血。

3. 动、静脉导管及三通，均要事先用肝素溶液充盈并排除空气。

4. 实验结束撤除动脉插管前，先将颈总动脉和股动脉结扎再拔管。

【思考题】

1. 实验过程中动物血压的变化趋势如何？分析其具体机制。

2. 血液回推后，血压可能恢复不到失血前的水平，为什么？如何处理？

（赵利军　门秀丽）

Experiment 22　Hemorrhagic shock

[**Experimental objectives**]　To duplicate the animal model of hemorrhagic shock; to observe manifestations of the animal in hemorrhagic shock, especially the change of BP, and to understand the pathogenesis.

[**Experimental principles**]　Occurrence of hemorrhagic shock depends on the speed and volume of blood loss. In this experiment, more than 30% of the total volume of blood will be exsanguinated quickly. The decrease of effective circulating blood volume excites sympathetic nerve reflectively. Then peripheral vessels constrict, causing rapid reduction of microcirculation perfusion, and leading to shock.

[**Experimental object**]　rabbit

[**Experimental materials**]　BL－420, 25% urethane, heparin solution, surgical instruments, syringe (5 ml, 50 ml), artery cannula (2), tracheal cannula, intravenous cannula, three-way pipe (3), arterial clamp, surgical thread, gauze

[**Experimental procedures**]

1. Preoperative preparation　Weigh the rabbit and anaesthetize it with 25% urethane (4 ml/kg) via the marginal vein of the ear to induce a general anaesthesia. Fix it in a dorsal position on the operating table. Shear the hair of the neck and groin.

2. Neck surgery　Cut the skin along the midline. Separate the trachea, and conduct tracheal intubation. Separate one side carotid artery. Inject heparin via an ear vein. Then perform carotid artery intubation with the three-way pipe connected to BL－420 for recording arterial blood pressure. Separate an external jugular vein and conduct venous intubation.

3. Observation on the normal state　Record the normal blood pressure (BP), heart rate (HR), respiratory rate (RR), color of skin and mucous.

4. Bloodletting　Separate one side thigh artery and conduct thigh artery cannulation. Connect the heparin rinsed 50 ml sterile syringe with the three-way pipe, and exsanguinate blood until BP drop to 1/3 of normal. Observe the changes of the indications during the procedure of bloodletting.

5. Rescue　When BP further drops with decompensation, infuse the blood back via venous cannula. And observe the changes of indexes.

[**Observational items**]

Blood pressure (BP), heart rate (HR), respiratory rate (RR), color of skin and mucous

[**Precautions**]

1. Depth of anesthesia should be moderate. Too shallow anesthesia may cause neurogenic shock by severe pain; deep anesthesia may inhibit respiration.

2. Avoid accidental hemorrhage during surgery.

3. Arterial cannula, intravenous cannula and the three-way pipe should be filled with heparin solution before use.

4. Remember to ligate the vessels before withdrawing the cannula.

[**Questions**]

1. What are the different changes at different stages of hemorrhagic shock? And analyze the pathogenesis.

2. BP may not recover to the pre-hemorrhage level. What's the reason? And how can you deal it?

(Wu Jing   Men Xiuli)

实验二十三　　急性右心衰竭

【实验目的】　掌握急性右心衰竭动物模型的复制方法；观察急性右心衰竭时动物的表现，并分析其发生机制。

【实验原理】　负荷过度是引起心力衰竭的重要原因，心脏各腔室负荷过度的常见原因各异。本实验通过耳缘静脉缓慢注入栓塞剂液体石蜡，引起肺动脉高压，即右心室后负荷加大。再经颈静脉输入大量生理盐水，增加右心室的前负荷。在前、后负荷急剧增加的情况下，右心室的收缩和舒张功能降低，导致急性右心衰竭。全身性静脉淤血、组织缺氧及水肿是右心衰的主要表现，通过相关指标观察机体的变化。

【实验对象】　家兔

【实验用品】　兔台，BL－420 生物机能实验系统，25％乌拉坦溶液，液体石蜡，水浴锅，手术器械，肝素，注射器（2 ml，5 ml，20 ml），动脉导管，静脉导管，三通（2 个），气管插管，动脉夹，输液装置，手术线，纱布

【实验步骤】

1. 麻醉固定　取兔一只并称重，25％乌拉坦（4 ml/kg）耳缘静脉缓慢注射麻醉动物，将其仰卧位固定于兔台，颈部剪毛。

2. 颈部手术　沿颈正中线剪开皮肤 6～7 cm，钝性分离颈部肌肉暴露气管，分离气管并做气管插管。分离一侧颈总动脉及另一侧颈外静脉并穿线备用。耳缘静脉注入肝素 1 ml/kg（1000 U/kg）。结扎颈总动脉远心端，动脉夹夹闭其近心端，在阻断血流段靠近头端 1/3 处用眼科剪剪一小口，将动脉插管插入并固定。打开三通，观察有无血压波动曲线。

3. 建立输液通路　连接输液装置，以 80 ml/kg 的量向输液瓶中注入生理盐水，排除管道中的气泡。通过颈静脉插管，缓慢滴注少量生理盐水以维持静脉通路。

4. 正常状态的观察　观察并记录家兔正常状态下的血压、心率、呼吸。

5. 增加右心后负荷　用注射器抽取预先水浴加热至 38 ℃的液体石蜡 0.5 ml/kg，经耳缘静脉缓慢注入，直至动脉血压下降 10～30 mmHg，观察并记录各项指标的变化。

6. 增加右心前负荷　待动物呼吸、血压稳定后，以 60～80 滴/min 的速度经颈静脉插管输入生理盐水。密切观察各项指标的变化，直至动物死亡。

7. 解剖观察　动物死亡后，挤压胸壁，观察气管内有无分泌物溢出，注意其性状。剖开胸、腹腔，观察有无胸水、腹水，肝体积及外观情况，肠壁有无水肿，肠系膜血管充盈情况。

【观察项目】　急性右心衰前后动物血压、心率、呼吸、皮肤黏膜颜色、全身性水肿情况（表 4－13）。

表 4-13 急性右心衰发生过程中各观察指标的变化记录表
Tab. 4-13 Changes of the indicators during acute right heart failure

观察时间 Time	心率（次/min） HR	血压（mmHg） BP	呼吸（次/min） RR	皮下水肿 Cutaneous dropsy	发绀 Cyanosis
正常 Normal					
注射液体石蜡后 After infusion of paraffin					
注射生理盐水后 After infusion of saline					

【注意事项】

1. 注入液体石蜡时一定要缓慢，否则动物极易因急性肺栓塞而迅速死亡。

2. 若生理盐水输液量超过 200 ml/kg，而各项指标变化仍不显著时，可再补充注入栓塞剂。

3. 解剖过程中不要损伤胸腹壁大血管，以免影响对胸腹水的观察。

【思考题】

1. 本实验动物出现急性右心衰的原因和机制是什么？

2. 实验过程中动物有无缺氧？缺氧的类型及发生机制是什么？

（赵利军　门秀丽）

Experiment 23　Acute right heart failure

[**Experimental objectives**]　To duplicate the animal model of acute right heart failure in rabbit; to observe manifestations of the animal, and to understand the pathogenesis.

[**Experimental principles**]　Pressure overload of the right heart is induced by slow injection of liquid paraffin via the marginal ear vein, which causes pulmonary embolism. Volume overload of the right heart is induced by infusing massive normal saline. Reduced systolic and diastolic functions of the right ventricle lead to acute right heart failure.

[**Experimental object**]　rabbit

[**Experimental materials**]　BL-420, 25% urethane, heparin solution, liquid paraffin, water bath, surgical instruments, syringe (2 ml, 5 ml, 20 ml), artery cannula, tracheal cannula, intravenous cannula, three-way pipe (2), arterial clamp, intravenous infusion device, surgical thread, gauze

[**Experimental procedures**]

1. Preoperative preparation　Weigh the rabbit and anaesthetize it with 25% urethane (4 ml/kg) via the marginal vein of the ear to induce a general anaesthesia. Fix it in a dorsal position on the operating table. Shear the hair of neck.

2. Neck surgery　Cut the skin along the midline. Separate the trachea, and perform tra-

cheal intubation. Separate one side carotid artery. Inject heparin via the marginal ear vein. Then conduct carotid artery intubation with the three-way pipe connected to BL – 420 for recording arterial blood pressure. Separate an external jugular vein and conduct venous intubation. Infuse normal saline at 5 – 10 drops/min.

3. Observation on the normal state　Record the normal blood pressure (BP), heart rate (HR), and respiratory rate (R)

4. Pressure overload of the right heart　Inject 0.5 ml/kg of 38 ℃ liquid paraffin via a marginal ear vein slowly, till BP decreases by 10 – 30 mmHg. Observe and record the changes.

5. Volume overload of the right heart　Infuse 80 ml/kg of saline at 60 – 80 drops/min till death.

6. Anatomical Observation　Squeeze the chest wall to observe whether there is outflow of overflow tracheal secretions. Open the chest and abdomen to observe whether there is pleural effusion, ascites, and intestinal wall edema. Observe the filling of mesenteric vessels, liver volume and appearance.

〔**Observations**〕　Blood pressure (BP), heart rate (HR), respiratory rate (R), color of skin and mucous, generalized edema.

〔**Precautions**〕

1. The liquid paraffin must be injected slowly, or severe pulmonary embolism may induce death.

2. If there is still no significant change of the indexes when the infusion volume of normal saline has been over 200 ml/kg, you should inject more liquid paraffin should be injected.

〔**Questions**〕

1. What are the cause and pathogenesis of acute right heart failure in this experiment?

2. Has the animal experienced hypoxia during the experiment? What's the type and pathogenesis of hypoxia?

(Wu Jing　Men Xiuli)

实验二十四　神经干动作电位的测定及麻醉药的影响

【实验目的】　学习蟾蜍（蛙类）坐骨神经-腓神经标本的制备方法；观察蟾蜍坐骨神经干复合动作电位的基本波形；了解神经纤维传导兴奋的特征；观察机械损伤及麻醉药对动作电位产生和传导的影响。

【实验原理】　神经纤维的兴奋表现为动作电位的产生和传导，神经纤维上传导的动作电位称为神经冲动。当神经纤维在某一点受到刺激产生兴奋时，组织兴奋的部位较未兴奋的或兴奋已恢复部位呈负电性，因此用电生理学方法可引导出此电位差。如果两个引导电极置于兴奋性正常的神经干表面，兴奋波先后通过两个电极处，便引导出两个方向相反的电位波形，称为双相动作电位。如果两个引导电极之间的神经纤维完全损伤，兴奋波只通过第一个引导电极，不能传至第二个引导电极，则只能引导出一个方向的电位波形，称为单相动作电位。坐骨神经干内含有无数条神经纤维，因此所记录的动作电位是一群阈值不同、传导速度不同、振幅不同的峰总和而成，称为复合动作电位。在一定范围内所记录的复合动作电位的幅值与刺激强度有关，即在阈刺激和最大刺激之间动作电位的幅值，随刺激强度的增加而递增。利多卡因可阻滞电压门控钠通道，影响动作电位的产生和传导而产生局部麻醉作用。

【实验对象】 蟾蜍

【实验用品】 蛙类手术器械一套，神经屏蔽盒，电极，BL－420 生物机能实验系统，培养皿，滴管，烧杯，纱布，棉线，林格液，2％盐酸利多卡因注射液

【实验步骤】

1. 破坏脑和脊髓 取蟾蜍一只，用自来水冲去泥沙。左手持蟾蜍使头前屈，右手握探针，从枕骨大孔垂直刺入，然后向前刺入颅腔并左右搅动捣毁脑组织，再将探针向椎管内刺入破坏脊髓，此时如动物四肢松弛，呼吸停止，表示破坏完全。

2. 剪除躯干上部及内脏 在骶髂关节上方约 1～1.5 cm 处用粗剪刀剪断脊柱，并沿其两侧剪除内脏及头胸部，仅保留后肢、骶骨及脊柱下半部。

3. 剥皮 用镊子夹住脊柱断端（不要夹住或接触神经），右手捏紧皮肤边缘，向下撕掉全部后肢的皮肤，然后将标本放入盛有林格液的培养皿中。将手和用过的器械洗净擦干。

4. 分离两后肢 用粗剪刀剪除尾骨后沿正中线将两条后肢和脊柱剪开（注意勿损伤坐骨神经），将分离的两条后肢放入盛有林格液的培养皿中。

5. 游离神经 取蟾蜍一条后肢背侧固定于蛙板上，循股二头肌和半膜肌之间的坐骨神经沟，用玻璃分针纵向分离出坐骨神经股骨段直至腘窝。在坐骨神经由脊柱发出的部位用丝线结扎并在近脊柱侧用眼科剪剪断神经。轻提结扎线，剪断坐骨神经的所有小分支，游离出坐骨神经。在腘窝处，用眼科剪剪断胫神经，继续向下分离走行于小腿肌肉表面的腓神经至踝关节，用丝线结扎后在其远端剪断，游离出坐骨神经-腓神经标本。游离出的神经干标本浸入林格液中 5～15 min，使其兴奋性稳定。

6. 连接实验装置 取一神经干标本小心搭在神经屏蔽盒内的刺激电极和引导电极上，确认神经与各电极接触良好，屏蔽盒接地线。将电极连接于 BL－420 生物机能实验系统相应位置，如图 4－10 所示。打开 BL－420 生物机能实验系统，开始实验。

【观察项目】

1. 启动刺激器（刺激方式为单刺激，刺激强度为 0～2 V，波宽 0.05 ms）刺激神经标本，记录正常复合动作电位。观察神经干复合动作电位的幅度在一定范围内随刺激强度变化而变化的现象，并得出阈刺激和最大刺激。

2. 将整个神经干标本方向倒置后，观察双相动作电位波形有无变化。

3. 在刺激电极与记录电极之间滴 1 滴 2％利多卡因（要在神经干上附着，以便充分作用），然后每隔 1 min 刺激几秒钟并记录，直至动作电位明显减小。

4. 用林格液冲洗恢复 15 min 后，分别在两记录电极之间以及刺激电极与记录电极之间剪断神经，观察刺激时动作电位的波形变化。

【注意事项】

1. 操作中注意保护神经；为防止神经干燥应向屏蔽盒中加入少量林格液，并常向标本滴加林格液；刺激强度应由弱至强，不可一下用过强的刺激，以免损伤神经。

2. 神经干两端的结扎线不准与电极和盒底部的林格液接触。

3. 尽量减小动作电位的刺激伪迹，这样更容易确定动作电位离开基线的起始点。

102

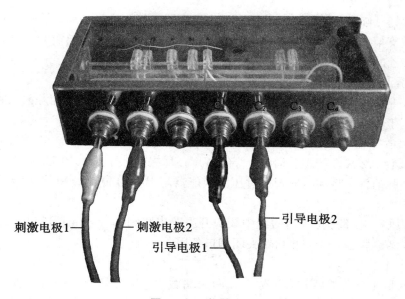

图 4 - 10　仪器连接

Fig. 4 - 10　Instrument connection

引导电极与 BL - 420 生物机能实验系统相应通道相连；两个刺激电极与刺激器相连

4. 禁止林格液打湿电极座。

【思考题】

1. 为什么一般情况下记录到双相动作电位的波形是不对称的？

2. 如何区别刺激伪迹与神经干动作电位？

3. 倒置神经干标本的放置方向的目的是什么？

4. 利多卡因对动作电位有何影响？为什么？

（王艳蕾）

实验二十五　麻醉期间不良刺激对循环功能的影响

【实验目的】　观察麻醉期间一些不良刺激对循环功能的影响，并分析其影响机制以及探讨消除不良影响的方法。

【实验原理】　麻醉对循环功能的影响取决于麻醉药的应用、通气方式、外科手术类别、失血量以及其他许多因素。许多全身麻醉药主要通过抑制交感神经系统的活动和压力感受器反射来影响循环功能，所以麻醉之后心血管代偿功能受到抑制，因不良刺激，如窒息、气管插管、腹腔探查、体位改变等所致的动脉血压的变化更为明显。这些不良刺激很容易刺激脏器的内脏神经（主要为迷走神经），导致异常的神经反射，引起心跳、血管舒缩及呼吸的变化，表现为血压、心率及呼吸的改变，严重者甚至出现心搏骤停及呼吸暂停。阿托品是 M 型胆碱能受体阻断剂，能防止因迷走神经传入引起的不良反射，进而消除各种不良刺激对循环功能的影响。

【实验对象】 家兔

【实验用品】 哺乳类动物手术器械，压力换能器，气管插管，动脉插管，兔手术台，丝线，纱布，铁支架，双凹夹，动脉夹，注射器，BL-420 生物机能实验系统，生理盐水，25％氨基甲酸乙酯，1000 U/ml 肝素，阿托品注射液

【实验步骤】

1. 麻醉、固定　家兔耳缘静脉缓慢注射 25％氨基甲酸乙酯（4 ml/kg）进行静脉麻醉后，仰卧固定于兔手术台上，剪去颈部手术部位的兔毛。

2. 分离气管　在颈部正中分离气管并穿线备用。

3. 动脉插管　分离左侧颈总动脉，穿线备用；耳缘静脉注射 1000 U/ml 肝素（1 ml/kg）后进行颈总动脉插管，将动脉插管通过压力换能器与 BL-420 生物机能实验系统相连，记录血压。

4. 暴露腹腔　腹部剪毛，沿腹正中线剪开腹壁皮肤约 3～5 cm 长切口，再沿腹白线剪开肌腱、腹膜暴露腹腔，先用止血钳夹闭切口备用。

【观察项目】

1. 在喉头以下气管处两软骨环之间，向头端做"⊥"形切口，进行气管内插管，观察血压的变化。

2. 堵住气管插管 15 s，阻塞呼吸道，观察血压的变化。

3. 分别取头高脚低位和脚高头低位，观察血压的变化。

4. 用力压迫兔双侧下颌深部区域的颈动脉窦，观察血压的改变。

5. 将肠管拉出腹腔外，进行腹腔探查，观察血压的变化。

6. 耳缘静脉注射 1 mg 阿托品，观察血压的变化，并于注射后第 1、第 5、第 8 min 再进行同样腹腔探查、气管插管，观察血压的变化。

【注意事项】

1. 整个实验过程中保持动脉插管与颈总动脉于平行位置，防止动脉插管刺破血管。

2. 每完成一个项目，需待血压恢复后，再进行下一项目的观察。

3. 腹腔探查时注意刺激强度保持一致。

【思考题】

1. 什么是不良刺激？在麻醉过程中观察这些不良刺激的影响对以后的工作有何意义？

2. 在麻醉过程中如何防止不良刺激对循环功能的影响？

（王艳蕾）

第五章　人体机能实验

实验一　人体动脉血压的测定及其影响因素

【实验目的】　掌握听诊法间接测量人体动脉血压的原理和方法；观察在正常情况下，运动和体位改变对动脉血压的影响，理解在不同生理条件下心血管活动的整合反应。

【实验原理】　血压是指流动着的血液对单位面积血管壁的侧压力。测定动脉血压的方法有直接法和间接法两种，通常采用间接法测定人体动脉血压，即柯氏（Korotkoff）音听诊法。间接法测量动脉血压原理是用血压计的袖带在所测动脉外施加压力，根据血管音的变化来测定血压。通常血液在血管内以层流形式流动，听不到声音，但如果在血管外施加压力使血管变窄，则血液通过狭窄处形成湍流产生杂音。因此，用袖带在肘关节上方肱动脉处加压，当袖带内压超过收缩压时，动脉血流完全被阻断，此时用听诊器在肱动脉迫处下方听不到任何声音，也触不到肱动脉的搏动。随后徐徐放气减小袖带内压，当袖带内压等于或略低于收缩压时，有少量血液通过肱动脉受压处，在其远侧血管内形成湍流产生杂音，此时在肱动脉的远端听到声音并触到脉搏，此时袖带内压力的读数为收缩压。若继续放气，随着袖带内压力的降低，通过肱动脉的血流量越多，血流持续时间越长，声音越来越强而变得清晰。当袖带内压力等于或稍低于舒张压时，血管处于张开状态，血流由湍流变为层流，声音突然降低或消失，此时袖带内压力的读数为舒张压。

人体运动时，交感神经系统活动加强，心率加快，心肌收缩力增强，心输出量增大，外周阻力增加，血压升高。体位改变时，由于重力作用使静脉回心血量发生改变，从而导致血压和心率的变化。

【实验对象】　人体

【实验用品】　血压计，听诊器

【实验步骤】

1. 熟悉听诊器和血压计的结构　听诊器由耳件和胸件两部分组成（图5-1）。血压计由检压计、袖带和橡皮球三部分组成。检压计是一个标有刻度的玻璃管（0～260 mmHg），上端与大气相通，下端与水银槽相通；袖带是一个外包布套的长方形橡皮囊，借助两根橡皮管分别与检压计的水银槽和橡皮球相连。橡皮球是一个带有螺丝帽的球状橡皮囊，供充气和放气用（图5-2）。

2. 动脉血压的测量

（1）受试者脱去一臂衣袖，静坐桌旁5 min。

（2）松开血压计上橡皮球的螺丝帽，将袖带内的空气完全排出，然后将螺丝帽旋紧，打开水银槽开关。

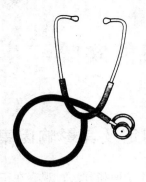

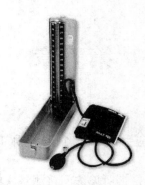

图 5-1　听诊器
Fig. 5-1　Stethoscope

图 5-2　血压计
Fig. 5-2　Sphygmomanometer

（3）受试者前臂平放于桌上，手掌向上，使上臂中心与心脏位置等高，将袖带缠于此上臂，袖带下缘距肘关节约 2 cm，松紧适宜（以能插入两指为宜）。

（4）将听诊器两耳件塞入检测者外耳道，务必使耳件的弯曲方向与外耳道一致。

（5）检测者在肘窝内侧先用手指触及肱动脉搏动处，然后将听诊器胸件置于其上。

（6）右手持橡皮球，向袖带内打气加压，同时听诊血管声音的变化，在声音消失后再加压 20～30 mmHg。随即慢慢松开橡皮球螺丝帽，徐徐放气，降低袖带内压，同时仔细听诊。在听到"嘣嘣"样第一声清晰而短促声音时，血压计上所示水银柱高度即代表收缩压。继续缓慢放气，这时声音先依次增强，后又逐渐减弱，最后完全消失。在声音突然由强变弱（或声音消失）这一瞬间，血压计上所示水银柱高度即代表舒张压。

【观察项目】

1. 正常动脉血压　受试者取坐位，保持安静状态，测量此体位的动脉血压。

2. 不同体位的动脉血压　受试者分别取卧位和站位，测量此两种体位时的动脉血压，并比较三种体位时的血压值。

3. 运动后的动脉血压　让受试者做原地蹲起运动，1 min 内完成 30 次，共做 2 min。分别测量运动后即刻、3 min 和 5 min 的血压。

【注意事项】

1. 室内保持安静以利于听诊。

2. 受试者右心房、上臂与血压计应保持同一水平面；袖带缠绕不能太紧或太松；听诊器的胸件压在肱动脉上要松紧适宜，切勿塞在袖带下进行测定。

3. 如血压超出正常范围，让受试者休息 10 min 后重复测量。

4. 正确使用血压计，充气前打开水银柱根部的开关，使用完毕后关上开关，以免水银溢出；同时将袖带内气体驱尽、卷好、放置盒内。

5. 重复测定时，袖带内压力必须降至 0 后再打气。

【思考题】

1. 影响动脉血压测定的因素有哪些？

2. 测量肱动脉血压时为什么上臂中心应与心脏在同一水平面？

3. 测量血压时为什么听诊器的胸件不能置于袖带下面？

（王艳蕾）

106

Experiment 1　Measurement and influence factors of the blood pressure in human

[Experimental objectives]　To study the method and principles of indirect blood pressure measurement in human; to observe the effects of posture change and sports on blood pressure.

[Experimental principles]　There are two kinds of methods to measure arterial blood pressure in human: direct measurement and indirect measurement. The indirect method is based on the correlation between blood pressure and arterial sound. An inflatable rubber bladder within a cloth cuff is wrapped around the upper arm, and a stethoscope is applied over the brachial artery. Initially, the cuff is usually inflated to produce a pressure greater than the systolic pressure so that the arterial blood flow is blocked, and no sound can be heard through stethoscope. The pressure in the cuff is read from an attached meter called sphygmomanometer. A valve is then turned to release air from the cuff, causing a gradual decrease in cuff pressure. When the cuff pressure is equal to or slightly more than the systolic pressure, the first Korotkoff sound is heard as blood passes in turbulent flow through the compressed artery. Korotkoff sound will continue to be heard during systole, as long as the cuff pressure remains greater than the diastolic pressure. When the cuff pressure becomes equal to or less than the diastolic pressure, the sound disappears because the artery remains open and laminar flow resumes. The last Korotkoff sound thus occurs when the cuff pressure is equal to the diastolic pressure.

Sports change and posture can affect the sympathetic tone and venous return, and then change the blood pressure.

[Experimental object]　human body

[Experimental materials]　sphygmomanometer, stethoscope

[Experimental procedures]

1. The structure of sphygmomanometer and stethoscope

Stethoscope is composed of two parts: earpieces and endpiece (Fig. 5 - 1). Sphygmomanometer consists of three parts: manometer, a cloth cuff and a rubber ball. The manometer is a glass tube that is marked with a scale of 0 - 260 mmHg. The upper end is opened to the atmosphere; the other end is communicated with a mercury groove. There is an inflatable rubber bladder within the cloth cuff. The cuff is communicated with a rubber ball and the mercury groove of manometer by rubber tubes. The rubber ball is a ball with a valve for deflation and inflation (Fig. 5 - 2).

2. Measurement of blood pressure

(1) The volunteer takes off a sleeve, and sits down calmly beside the table for more than 5 min.

(2) The volunteer lays the forearm on the table with the palm upwards, keeping the height of the upper arm equal to the position of the heart. Wind the cuff on the upper arm with proper tightness. The lower edge of the cuff should be 2 cm above the elbow joint at least.

(3) Loosen the screw valve on the rubber ball, expand the cuff and squeeze out the air from the cuff, and then close the valve.

(4) Place both earpieces of stethoscope in the external auditory canals; keep the curvature of the earpieces concordant with that of external auditory canals.

(5) Touch the pulse point of the brachial artery in the elbow fossa, and then put the endpiece of the stethoscope there.

(6) Use the rubber ball to pump air into the cuff. The mercury column in the glass tube rises gradually. When no sound can be heard from the stethoscope, stop pumping air (generally near to 180 mmHg). The valve is then turned to release air from the cuff, causing a gradual decrease in cuff pressure. When the first Korotkoff sound is heard, the height of the mercury column represents the systolic pressure. Continue to release air from the cuff. When the sound disappears or changes from strong to weak suddenly, the height of the mercury column represents the diastolic pressure.

[**Observations**]

1. Arterial blood pressure in calm status　The volunteer sits down beside the table calmly, and the blood pressure is measured in this position.

2. Arterial blood pressure in different position　The volunteer takes lying posture and standing posture, measure the blood pressure is measured in those two positions and blood pressure of the above three positions is compared.

3. Arterial blood pressure after sport　The volunteer squats down and stands up 2 min with the frequency of once every two seconds, and the blood pressure is measured at 0 min, 3 min and 5 min after sport respectively.

[**Precautions**]

1. Keep the room quiet to facilitate auscultation.

2. The position of the upper arm and the heart should be at the same level. The tightness of the inflated cuff should be proper. Stethoscope should be applied with light pressure to the brachial artery (heavy pressure will distort the artery and produce sound below the true diastolic pressure) and cannot be placed under the cuff.

3. If blood pressure is beyond the normal range, re-measure blood pressure after the volunteer has had a rest for 10 min.

4. Use the sphygmomanometer correctly. Open the switch before inflating the cuff, and close it after measurement in case that the mercury flows out.

5. Completely deflate the cuff before measurement.

[**Questions**]

1. What factors can affect the measurement of arterial blood pressure?

2. Why should the position of the upper arm and the heart be at the same level when the blood pressure is being measured?

3. Explain why the stethoscope cannot be placed under the cuff when measuring blood pressure?

(Wang Yanlei)

实验二　视野的测定

【实验目的】　学习视野的测定方法，并了解测定视野的意义。

【实验原理】　视野是单眼固定注视前方一点时所能看到的空间范围。正常人的视野范围，鼻侧和额侧较窄，颞侧与下侧较宽。除了解剖结构，许多因素可以影响视野，如视野中物体的移动性、物体的照明、物体的大小和物体的颜色。在相同亮度下，白色视野最大，红色次之，绿色最小。

测定视野有助于了解视网膜、视觉传导道和视觉中枢的功能，对一些疾病如青光眼、累及视神经的肿瘤等的早期诊断、制订治疗方案和病情判断具有重要意义。

【实验对象】　人体

【实验用品】　视野计，各色（白、红、黄或蓝、绿）视标，视野图纸，铅笔

【实验步骤】

1. 观察视野计的结构

最常用的是弧形视野计（图5-3）。它是一个安在支架上的半圆弧形金属板，可绕水平轴旋转360°。圆弧上有刻度为0~90，表示由该点射向视网膜周边的光线与视轴之间的夹角。视野界限即以此角度表示。圆弧一端与刻度盘一起固定在支架上，刻度盘上的刻度为0~180，其对面的支架上附有可上下移动的托颌架，托颌架上方附有眼眶托，测定时附着于受试者眼窝下方。此外，视野计附有各色视标，测定各种颜色的视野时使用。

2. 在明亮的光线下，受试者下颌放在托颌架上，眼眶下缘靠在眼眶托上，调整托架高度，使眼与弧架的中心点位于同一条水平线上。遮住一眼，另一眼注视弧架的中心点，接受测试。

3. 实验者从周边向中央慢慢移动弧架上白色的视标架，随时询问受试者是否看到视标，当受试者回答看到时，记录度数；再把视标从中央往周边慢慢移动，直到看不见为止，记录度数。求出这两点度数的平均值，并标注在视野图纸的相应经纬度上。用同样的方法测出弧架对侧的数值，也标记在视野图纸上。

4. 将弧架依次转动45°角，重复上述测定，共操作4次得出8个度数（0°，45°，90°，135°，225°，270°和315°），将视野图上8个点依次相连，便得出白色视野的范围，如图5-4所示。

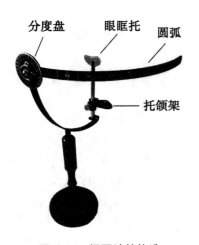

图5-3　视野计的构造

Fig. 5-3　The structure of perimeter

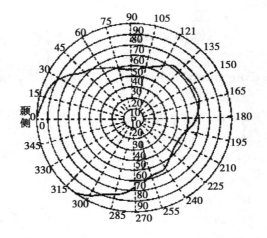

图5-4　左眼白色视野图

Fig. 5-4　The figure of white visual field in the left eye

109

5. 按上述方法分别测出该侧眼的红色、绿色视野。

6. 同法测出另一眼的白色、红色、绿色视野。将所得视野图数据填入下表。

视野图数据
Retinal mapping data

角度		0	45	90	135	180	225	270	315
白色可见	White in								
白色不可见	White out								
平均值	White mean								
红色可见	Red in								
红色不可见	Red out								
平均值	Red mean								
绿色可见	Green in								
绿色不可见	Green out								
平均值	Green mean								

【注意事项】

1. 测试视野时，受试者一定要固定注视弧架中心的镜子，不能随着视标的移动而移动，否则测得的视野偏大。

2. 受试者不应是色盲患者，要摘掉隐形眼镜。

3. 测试视野时，以受试者确实看到视标为准，受试者如果猜测，则放弃测试结果。

【思考题】

1. 什么叫视野？影响视野的因素有哪些？

2. 分析视网膜、视觉传导路和视觉中枢机能发生障碍时对视野的影响。

（杨秀红　耿　菲）

Experiment 2　Determination of visual field

[**Experimental objectives**]　To study the method of measuring visual field and to understand the significance of it.

[**Experimental principles**]　Visual field is the entire area seen by one eye when it is fixed forward at a certain point. On the medial or nasal side, the vision field is less than that on the temporal side due to presence of the bridge of nose. On the upper side, the vision field is less than that on the lower side due to obstruction by the superciliary arches.

In addition to the anatomy structure, many factors affect the visual field, such as mobility of the object in the visual field, illumination of the object, size of the object and color of the object. Under the same illumination, the visual field of different color is different in size: white>red>blue>green.

110

Determination of visual field helps to understand functions of retina, vision conduction and optic center. The visual field examination is important in the diagnosis and assessment of various diseases or conditions including glaucoma and those neurological diseases which affect the eyes, the optic nerve or the brain.

[**Experimental object**]　human body

[**Experimental materials**]　perimeter, perimetry markers of different colors, perimeter chart, pencil

[**Experimental procedures**]

1. The structure of perimeter

The perimeter consists of a semicircular metallic arc. This arc can be rotated on a pilot in any direction along with the test object. This arc is marked with the degree from 0 to 90, which will give the extent of the visual field. On the back of this arc, there are graduated markings going from 0 to 180. There are also some perimetry markers of different colors for use with the perimeter (Fig. 5 - 3).

2. The volunteer seats at the perimeter apparatus with the jaw on the hold for submaxilla, and stares at the central white spot. He/she is asked to cover the left eye with the left hand. Stare straight ahead and identify the color of the disk approaching from the periphery.

3. The experimenter picks a colored disk at random, and shows it to the data collector but not to the volunteer. Set the perimeter to the angle of approach to be tested. The experimenter moves the disk slowly and steadily along the arm from 90 degrees toward the central point (0 degree), and stops when the volunteer correctly reports the color. (The data collector should read the degrees from centre and record the degrees as the 'in' measure.)

4. This procedure is repeated and the disk is steadily moved outward until the subject reports no longer being able to see the color. (The data collector should record the degrees from centre as the 'out' measure.)

5. All the angles marked on the data sheet are to be tested. The experimenter moves both inward and outward using the white, red and green disks. Then the arc is rotated again for the other angles. Visual angles used are 0, 45, 90, 135, 180, 225, 270 and 315.

[**Precautions**]

1. Subject should not move his or her eyes side ways during testing.

2. Subject should not be color blind, nor wear contact lenses.

3. Subject should close the other eye. Do not guess the color.

[**Questions**]

1. What is visual field? What are the factors that affect the visual field?

2. Analyze the effects of dysfunction in retina, vision conduction and optic center on visual field.

(Yang Xiuhong　Daniel H. Nissen)

实验三　人体听力的检查和声音的传导途径

【实验目的】　通过音叉测试听力，了解并比较声波空气传导和骨传导的途径及其特征；学习临床上鉴别传音性耳聋和感音性耳聋的常用方法。

【实验原理】　声音传入耳蜗有两条途径：①气导：声波经外耳道引起鼓膜振动，再经听骨链和卵圆窗膜进入耳蜗；②骨导：声波直接引起颅骨振动，进而引起位于颞骨骨质中的耳蜗内淋巴液的振动。

正常生理状态下以空气传导为主，气导时程比骨导时程持续时间长，即林纳试验阳性；当气导的传音通路受阻时，气导时程缩短，等于或小于骨导时程，即林纳试验阴性。

正常情况下，人的两耳感受声波的功能相同；骨传导的敏感性比空气传导低得多，故在正常听觉中引起的作用甚微。但当鼓膜或中耳病变引起传音性耳聋时（或其他原因导致外耳至中耳的传音受损时），气导明显受损，而骨导却不受影响，甚至相对增强。将振动的音叉柄垂直压在被检查者前额正中发际处，听力正常时，两耳所感觉到的音叉音的强度是一样的，称为韦伯实验阳性。

临床上，由于鼓膜或中耳病变等空气传导障碍引起的听力下降或消失，称为传音性耳聋。由耳蜗等病变引起的听力下降或消失，称为感音性耳聋。

【实验对象】　人体

【实验用品】　音叉，棉球和橡皮锤

【实验步骤】

1. 比较同侧耳的气导和骨导（任内试验，图 5-5A）

（1）保持室内安静，受试者取坐位。

（2）检查者敲响音叉后，立即置音叉柄于受试者被检测的颞骨乳突部；当受试者刚刚听不到声音时，立即将振动的音叉置于受试者外耳道口 1 cm 处，两叉臂末端应与外耳道口在同一平面。受试者感觉声音的强弱及其变化。

（3）检查者敲响音叉后，先将振动的音叉置于受试者外耳道口 1 cm 处，两叉臂末端应与外耳道口在同一平面；当受试者刚刚听不到声音后立即将音叉柄置于受试者的颞骨乳突部。受试者感觉声音的强弱及其变化。

（4）用棉球塞住受试者外耳道（相当于空气传导途径受阻），重复上述操作。

2. 比较两耳的骨传导（韦伯试验，图 5-5B）

（1）敲击音叉后将叉柄底部紧压于颅顶中线上任何一点（或前额正中发际处），受试者两耳同时感受声音的强弱。

（2）用棉球塞住受试者一侧外耳道，重复上述操作，受试者两耳同时感受声音的强弱，记录两耳感受到的声音变化或受试者感到声音偏向哪一侧。

（3）取出棉球，将胶管一端塞入受试者某

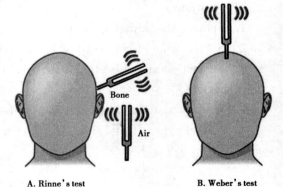

A. Rinne's test　　　　　　B. Weber's test

图 5-5　任内试验和韦伯试验示意图

Fig. 5-5　Rinne's test and Weber's test

一耳孔，胶管的另一端塞入另一个人的某侧耳孔，检查者将发音的音叉置于受试者同侧的颞骨乳突部，观察另一个人能否听到声音。

【观察项目】

1. 任内试验

（1）骨导检测无声后，再进行气导检测，受试者的听力情况如何？

（2）气导检测无声后，再进行骨导检测，受试者的听力情况如何？

2. 韦伯试验

（1）敲击音叉后，将叉柄底部紧压于颅顶中线上任何一点，受试者的听力情况如何？

（2）棉球塞住受试者一侧外耳道，敲击音叉后，将叉柄底部紧压于颅顶中线上任何一点，受试者的听力情况如何？

（3）胶管连接两受试者的左右耳，敲击音叉后置于一受试者插胶管侧颞骨乳突上，另一受试者感觉是否有声？

【注意事项】

1. 敲击音叉时，用力不可过猛，切忌在坚硬物品上敲击以防损害音叉，可在手或大腿上敲击。

2. 音叉放在外耳道口时，叉支的振动方向正对外耳道口，两者相距 1 cm，防止音叉叉支触及耳郭、皮肤及毛发。

【思考题】

1. 声波通过哪些途径传入内耳？为何正常情况下空气传导效果远高于骨传导？

2. 如何用实验鉴别传音性耳聋和感音性耳聋？

（杨秀红）

Experiment 3　Sound conduction tests

[**Experimental objectives**]　To compare air conduction with bone conduction; to learn how to distinguish conductive hearing loss from sensorineural hearing loss by sound conduction test.

[**Experimental principles**]　There are two ways in which sound is conducted into the inner ear: air conduction and bone conduction. Air conduction is the atmospheric transmission of sound to the inner ear through the external auditory canal and structures of the middle ear. Bone conduction is the conduction of sound waves to the cochlea through the cranial bones.

Normally, air conduction is the main way in which sound is conducted from the external ear into the cochlea. Air conduction is greater than bone conduction in normal people. So the conductive deafness and sensory neural (or perceptive) deafness can be defined by comparing those two conduction ways. Tuning fork tests give the information about the better hearing ear and type of deafness as well.

[**Experimental object**]　human body

[**Experimental materials**]　tuning fork, cotton ball, rubber hammer

[**Experimental procedures**]

1. Rinne's test　Bone conduction and air conduction of the same ear is compared (Fig. 5 - 5A).

(1) Vibrating tuning fork is placed on the mastoid process and when not heard, it is transferred immediately in the front of external auditory meatus. If not heard, this indicates that the bone conduction is more than air conduction or equivalent. To be more certain, this test is repeated in reverse order. Now tuning fork is placed against the pinna and when the subject can not hear sound, it is placed at the mastoid process. If air conduction is more than bone conduction, the subject would not be able to hear. But if bone conduction increases, the subject would hear it.

Normal: Air conduction is greater than bone conduction, Rinne's positive.

Conductive deafness: Bone conduction is greater than air conduction, Rinne's negative.

Sensory - neural deafness: Air conduction is greater than bone conduction (because both air conduction and bone conduction are equivalently decreased), Rinne's positive.

(2) "Rinne's false negative" is found in the case of severe sensory neural deafness in one ear. In this situation, Weber's test will lateralize in the normal ear instead of lateralizing in the ear in which initially Rinne's test was positive.

2. Weber's test　Bone conduction of both ears is compared (Fig. 5 - 5B).

Footplate of the vibrating tuning fork is placed in the center of the vertex or forehead and the subject is asked to answer that in which ear he listens better. If he answers that he listens equally in both ears, then it is said that Weber's test is central which means that either he is normal or having the same degree and type of deafness on both sides. If he answers that he listens better in one ear then it is said that Weber's test is lateralized in that ear. Normally it should lateralize in the ear in which initially Rinne's test was negative.

[**Precautions**]

1. Knock the tuning fork with your palm gently.

2. Hold the tuning fork by the base shaft with your fingers, but do not allow the fork end to come in contact with other objects such as hair or skin.

[**Questions**]

1. How many auditory conductive pathways do people have? Please explain their routes?

2. How to distinguish the conductive deafness from sensorineural deafness by tests?

(Yang Xiuhong)

第六章 设计性实验

第一节 概 述

设计性实验又称探索性实验，是在生理学、病理生理学、药理学等医学基础课和文献检索、医学统计学、实验动物学等课程的基础上构建的一门综合性实践课程。系指采用科学的逻辑思维配合实验方法和技术，对拟定研究的目的（或问题）进行的一种有明确目的的探索性研究。

第二节 实验选题

著名科学家爱因斯坦曾经指出："提出一个问题往往比解决一个问题更重要，因为解决一个问题也许仅仅是一个数学上或实验上的技能而已。而提出新的问题、新的可能性，以新的角度去看旧的问题，却需要创造性的想象力，而且标志着科学的真正进步。"因此，选择课题是科学研究中具有战略意义的首要问题。选题要从程序上做到先积累资料、选题意向和查新，而后确认选题方向和立题。

一、实验选题的基本原则

1. 创新性 选题必须具有创新性，包括提出新规律、新技术、新方法或对原有规律、技术、方法的补充和改进。

2. 科学性 课题的选择要以科学思想为指导，以事实为依据。即选题要有理论基础和实践基础。

3. 实用性 是指通过该设计性实验可以解决医学实践中存在的实际问题。

4. 可行性 选题要充分考虑到影响实验实施的各种主、客观因素和条件。

二、实验选题的基本过程

（一）提出问题

科学问题的选择不是一个简单的过程，而是一门艺术。科学问题的来源可以通过如下渠道来实现。

1. 实践积累中选题 根据以往的科研经历或临床实践经验进行选题。

2. 理论积累中选题 通过查阅大量感兴趣领域的文献，从中发现感兴趣的问题。

3. 学科的边缘交叉区选题 例如，基础性的课题要跟临床实践关联，而临床课题要通过基础的技术手段来证明，在各学科的边缘交叉区可以选择我们感兴趣的课题。

4. 移植和引用 同一系统的各个器官，类似疾病的研究指标和方法可以相互借鉴。例如，同为消化系统肿瘤的胃癌和肝癌，在某些发病机制或治疗手段上一定有可以相互借鉴之处。因此，研究肝癌时，可以借鉴胃癌的研究指标或方法等。

5. 从学术争论中选择课题　学术会议中有争论的问题同样可以作为研究课题。

6. 在各级项目中选题　各级项目申报指南中提出的一些资助重点和范围，基本都是关系国计民生的问题，如果把这些内容作为研究课题，则更具有实用性。

（二）查阅文献

有了科学问题之后，就要进行相关的文献检索。通过阅读相关文献，了解该课题的知识背景、国内外研究现状，发现目前该研究领域尚待解决的科学问题，确定最佳的研究方法和技术路线，并最终形成前沿的、高水平的研究题目。只有充分阅读相关的文献，才能在实验研究过程中避免重复前人工作，从而使课题能够顺利实施。

（三）形成假说

提出了科学问题并查阅了大量文献后，通过对所研究的问题进一步加工总结，最终升华成科学假说。例如，德国药物学家贝林在白喉的早期研究中发现，实验动物注射白喉杆菌死亡时，细菌仍留在注射点周围。那么，动物是由什么原因引起死亡的呢？他提出了细菌毒素是其原因的假说。

（四）完成标书

对科学问题形成假说并确定了课题题目后，必须对所选的课题进行全面、细致的陈述，并按照立题背景、研究内容、技术路线、预期实验结果等填写完整的标书。

三、选题范围参考

（一）对原有实验方法和技术的改进

例如，在原有实验方法和技术的基础上稍加修改，使其更加简便易行等。

（二）建立一种新的动物模型及评价该模型的指标

根据自己的科研经验建立一种新的动物模型，然后通过以下几个方面进行评价：①实验结果表达率高，而且稳定可靠；②可重复性好；③实验方法更趋于简单、实用；④能被多数学者承认、借用；⑤学术上解决了一些临床实际问题，而且有推广使用价值。

（三）探讨发病机制

例如神经递质、体液因子、生物介质、抗原、抗体、药物等的作用。

（四）研究某种药物的体内代谢过程或作用机制

（五）治疗某种疾病或病理过程的新方法、新技术

例如生物制品药物、生物物理学技术、核素制品等。

（秦丽娟）

第三节　实验设计

实验设计是研究者在实验前根据研究目的拟定的实验计划及方法策略，其主要内容是合理安排实验程序，并提出将如何对实验数据作统计学分析等。实验设计中需要注意如下一些问题。

一、基本要素

（一）处理因素
一般是指外加于受试对象，在实验中需要观察并阐明其处理效应的因素。
1. 物理因素　例如电、磁、光、声、温度、射线、力等处理因素。
2. 化学因素　例如药物、营养素、激素、毒物等化学物质。
3. 生物因素　例如寄生虫、真菌、细菌、病毒、生物制品等。

（二）受试对象
各种处理因素所针对的对象即为受试对象，例如实验用到的动物、细胞或临床标本等。

（三）实验效应
实验因素取不同水平时，在实验单位上所产生的反应称为实验效应。实验效应必须通过具体的指标来体现。应尽可能多地选用特异性强、灵敏度高、准确可靠的客观指标。

二、基本原则

（一）对照原则　设立空白对照组、实验对照组等。
（二）随机原则　运用"随机数字表"、"随机排列表"、"伪随机数"等实现随机化。
（三）重复原则　在相同实验条件下必须做多次独立重复实验。重复 5 次以上的实验才具有较高的可信度。

三、填写实验设计书（见下表）

实验设计书
Design of experimental scheme

实验设计书			
研究题目：			
理论依据及研究现状：			
研究内容：			
研究方法：			
实验对象：	性别：	规格：	数量：
实验组与对照组的处理：			
观察指标：			

实验步骤:
仪器与药品:
预期实验结果:
设计人:

四、开题报告与完善实验设计

将实验设计的内容向师生汇报，听取大家的评审意见后，集思广益，进而更好地修改与完善实验设计方案，最终形成高水平和高质量的实验设计。

（秦丽娟）

第四节　实验实施

完成实验设计书后，按照实验设计书的技术路线流程完成整个实验设计，具体包括如下过程。

一、实验准备

包括文献知识准备、实验动物及试剂耗材准备等。

二、预实验

正式实验之前，用标准物质或只用少量样品进行实验，以便摸索出最佳的实验条件，并加以优化，为正式实验奠定基础。

三、正式实验

根据预实验的实验条件和实验设计书，完全按照实验设计的步骤完成整个实验过程。在此过程中要做好实验记录，及时总结和分析实验结果，并动态追踪该领域的最新研究进展，对实验设计做必要的补充和修改。

四、数据收集、整理和分析

根据预先拟定的原始记录方式和内容记录文字、数据、表格、图形和图片。对原始数据整理成表，进行数据处理和统计学分析。

（秦丽娟）

第五节　医学科研论文撰写

一、概　述

医学科研论文是医学科研工作者在科研工作的基础上，将自己在实验中得到的第一手资料进行整理、归纳、分析而撰写的文章，是医学科研工作的重要内容。在一项医学科研活动结束后，总要用文字将整个活动过程和活动结果的具体内容描述出来，总结成文并公之于世，这是医学科研成果最普遍、也是不可缺少的一部分。

（一）医学科研论文的类型

一般医学刊物中刊用的文章，大致可分为以下几种类型：述评、论著、病例报告、临床病例讨论、学术交流、综述、专题笔谈、经验介绍、讲座和简讯等。

（二）医学科研论文的基本结构（以论著为例）

1. 题目（Title）　　题目是论文的总纲，是对论文内容的高度概括和综合，必须新颖、简洁，突出重点，紧扣文章内容，一般少于 25 字。

2. 作者（Author）　　论文作者只限于那些选定研究课题和制定研究方案，直接参加全部或主要部分研究工作并做出贡献，以及参加撰写论文并对内容负责的人，按其贡献大小排列名次。论文第一作者应是论文课题的创意者、设计者、执行者，是论文的执笔者。通讯作者一般是论文的指导老师或课题负责人。作者人数不宜过多，一般不超过 6 人。

3. 摘要（Abstract）　　论文摘要是论文的缩影，是全文的浓缩版。它高度概括了文章的所有主要信息，通常排在正文开始之前，可独立存在。摘要的撰写要求简明扼要，高度概括，格式规范，富有逻辑性，一般为 100～300 字。摘要按格式分为结构式摘要和资料性摘要。结构式摘要分目的（Objectives）、方法（Methods）、结果（Results）、结论（Conclusions）四部分撰写，分别冠以四个副标题；资料性摘要总结所有四部分的主要内容，写成完整段落而无副标题。英文摘要与中文摘要在意义上基本对应，包括文题、作者姓名（汉语拼音）、单位名称、所在城市名及邮政编码。

4. 关键词（Key words）　　关键词是医学论文的文献检索标识，是简明表达文献主题概念的语言词汇。一般 3～8 个，掌握"精、准、少"的原则。

5. 前言（Introduction）　　前言常采用从宽到窄的"漏斗式"结构，从一个比较大的研究领域引导到研究课题的专门领域，然后提出本文要解决的问题，即围绕提出问题的依据、解决问题的关键、重要性和意义进行简明扼要的说明。前言的字数一般为 200～500 字，约占全文的 1/8 或 1/10。

6. 材料与方法（Materials and methods）　　材料与方法是执行科研的关键部分，是判断论文科学性和先进性的主要依据，事关研究的质量，也是论文被拒的常见原因之一。根据论文性质以及期刊的要求，也可以改称为"资料与方法"、"对象与方法"、"病例和方法"等。主要内容包括实验对象与分组、实验仪器（名称、生产厂家、型号等）和材料（药品和试

119

剂）、实验的方法（观察的指标和检测方法等）以及统计学方法。

7. 结果（Results）　结果部分是一篇论文的心脏，是论文价值所在，是研究成果的结晶，全文结论由此得出，讨论由此引发，判断推理和建议由此导出。结果的表达方式主要有文字表述、表格、插图三种方式，选择哪一种方式来表达研究数据，取决于研究资料的类型。当数据较少或根据数据得出的结论较为简单宜采用文字表达方式；文字表述也可用于对数据、图表、照片的说明。插图包括示意图、曲线图、照片图等，要求大小比例适中，粗细均匀，数字清晰，照片黑白对比分明；每幅图都有图序和图题，写在图下。表格采用三线表格，一个典型的表格包括标题、专栏的分标题、数据和脚注四部分内容。

8. 讨论（Discussion）　讨论是论文的重要主体部分，也是论文中最难撰写的部分。讨论部分是详细解释作者的研究结果，并通过他人发表的研究结果衬托出作者的研究结果的重要意义，以及为将来的进一步研究提出建设性意见。忌重复叙述实验结果，或写成文献综述，应紧密结合自己的资料与结果，从理论上有选择地对研究结果进行分析、比较、解释和推理。

9. 参考文献（References）　参考文献是文献目录的一种特殊形式，载于正文之末，为撰写或编辑论文和著作而引用的有关文献信息资源，是作者经过精心挑选的与论文主题内容有密切关系的文献；在一定程度上能反映该篇论文的全部或部分观点，能对正文起到补充与佐证的作用。参考文献的著录格式可参考投稿杂志的投稿须知。

二、医学科研论文的撰写过程

（一）资料准备
资料的准备包括准备实验数据、结果、图表和文献等相关资料。

（二）撰写提纲
经过反复思考，理清思路，形成条目，写出提纲。提纲是论文的基本骨架，有了提纲，作者写起来就会目标明确，思路开通。提纲的内容主要是按题目、前言（文章的宗旨目的）、实验材料与方法、讨论与结论的顺序进行。

（三）写作成文
提纲拟定后，根据自己的思路，妥当安排内容的先后次序，然后将自己的观点充分表达。在写作初稿时，不妨内容写的全一些，面宽一些，避免有重要内容遗漏；而且最好能集中一段时间和精力，使文章一气呵成。

（四）修改完善
文章初稿完成后，应征求各方面的意见，尤其是共同的工作者与指导者，然后加以反复推敲并做细致的修改。文章全部完成后，最好放置一段时间，再行修改。"温故而知新"常可发现重要问题，因此需要多次修改。修改的重点是篇幅的压缩、结构的调整、语言和内容的修改等。

（五）投稿发表
文章修改完善后，选择合适的杂志进行投稿。当确定杂志后，必须认真阅读该杂志的"投稿须知"，严格按照投稿须知中的规定认真修改，例如字数的限制、文章内容的编排、图表制作的要求和参考文献引用的格式等。稿件投出后，要随时关注稿件处理情况。如果编辑部要求修稿，文章被录用的机会比较大；作者应根据审稿人和编辑部的意见，逐条进行修改和说明。最后，编辑部根据审稿专家对修改稿的意见，作出是否录用的决定。文章一旦被录用，经编辑部排版、校样，最后发表。

（王艳蕾）

第六节　设计性实验参考项目

设计性实验一　肾素-血管紧张素系统与心血管疾病

肾素-血管紧张素系统（Renin - angiotensin system，RAS）是体内重要的体液调节系统。目前认为，RAS 由多个酶、效应分子和受体组成，主要有肾素、血管紧张素原、血管紧张素转换酶（ACE）、血管紧张素转换酶 2（ACE2）、血管紧张素 Ⅱ 及其受体 AT1 和 AT2、血管紧张素（1-7）及其受体 Mas 等；它们共同作用于肾、血管等组织，主要功能是调节血压、水和电解质平衡及维持心血管稳态等。肾素-血管紧张素系统既存在于循环系统中，也存在于血管壁、心脏、中枢、肾和肺等组织中，共同参与对靶器官的调节。如果 RAS 失调，可导致血压升高，严重时伴随肾和心血管的损害。目前已有几十种血管紧张素转化酶抑制剂（ACEI）和血管紧张素受体阻断剂（ARBs），成为当前控制高血压、防治心肌肥厚等最有效的药物。RAS 系统中 ACE2、血管紧张素（1-7）等新成员的发现和对其生理意义的研究让我们对 RAS 有了许多新的认识，也促进了以 RAS 为靶标的新型抗高血压药物的研究。

本实验由学生根据课堂所学有关肾素-血管紧张素系统和血压的形成等理论知识，结合国内外相关研究，自行设计一个动物实验，使学生在巩固书本知识的同时，进一步开拓思维。在实验设计过程中，需考虑以下几个问题。

1. 高血压发病时 RAS 系统有何变化？
2. 高血压动物实验模型的种类及其研究进展。
3. 以 RAS 系统为靶标的药物都有哪些？临床评价如何？
4. 应用 RAS 系统药物进行动物实验，如何进行动物分组？选择哪种给药方法？观察哪些指标？

（杨秀红）

设计性实验二　缓激肽开放胶质瘤大鼠血脑屏障的作用及其可能机制

设计背景：神经胶质瘤在颅内各种肿瘤中最为多见。胶质瘤的治疗以手术治疗为主，但由于其可扩散至邻近或远离原发灶的脑组织，手术很难将肿瘤组织彻底切除。因此，术后进行化学治疗等极为必要。由于血脑屏障的存在，限制了各种大分子和小分子非脂溶性药物通过血脑屏障到达肿瘤组织。目前国内外研究发现，缓激肽可增加治疗药物进入胶质瘤组织，但其确切机制尚未完全明了。

提示：可以从生理学研究的三个水平来进行设计。

1. 整体水平：制备胶质瘤大鼠模型。

2. 器官和系统水平：经颈总动脉给予胶质瘤大鼠缓激肽后，再经尾静脉给予伊文思蓝，选取不同的时间点取出胶质瘤大鼠脑组织，观察缓激肽是否可以开放胶质瘤的血脑屏障（血脑屏障开放的脑组织呈蓝色，没有开放的脑组织不呈现蓝色）。

3. 细胞和分子水平：利用分子生物学方法检测给予缓激肽后的胶质瘤细胞中某种蛋白的改变情况，进而推测缓激肽开放胶质瘤血脑屏障的可能机制。

（秦丽娟）

设计性实验三　某药对肠道平滑肌活动的影响及机制探讨

消化道平滑肌具有自动节律性、较大的伸展性和紧张性，对化学物质（某些药物）、温度变化及牵张刺激较敏感等特性。小肠离体后，置于适宜环境中，仍能进行节律性的活动。肠管平滑肌上存在多种受体，如 M-胆碱能受体、肾上腺素能（α、β）受体、组胺受体以及 5-羟色胺受体等。不同受体兴奋时对肠平滑肌的作用不同，M 和 H 受体兴奋时，肠平滑肌收缩；α、β 受体兴奋时，肠平滑肌松弛。有些药物（$BaCl_2$）对肠平滑肌有直接兴奋作用，而阿托品对其无影响。小肠的纵行和环行肌层间有肌间神经丛，其末梢释放乙酰胆碱，作用于肠平滑肌的 M-胆碱受体，所以离体肠平滑肌在适当的营养液中仍能有节律地缓慢收缩与舒张，持续数小时。用动物的离体肠管可以分析药物对不同受体的兴奋和拮抗作用。

建议本实验由学生自己设计，观察某药对胃肠道活动的作用，并探讨可能的作用机制。从动物选择、分组、给药方法、观察指标等，证明某药对肠道平滑肌是否有影响，并从受体角度讨论分析其对肠平滑肌作用的可能机制。

（韩淑英）

设计性实验四　应激时动物机体的变化

应激是指机体在各种内外环境因素刺激时所出现的非特异性全身反应。引起应激或应激反应的各种刺激因素称为应激源，包括内、外环境和心理、社会因素。机体受到应激源刺激时，主要的神经-内分泌反应为蓝斑-交感-肾上腺髓质系统和下丘脑-垂体-肾上腺皮质系统的强烈兴奋，使血浆中儿茶酚胺和糖皮质激素含量明显增高，并由此引起生理、生化的变化和心理、行为的变化，包括三大营养物质的代谢改变和中枢神经系统、心血管系统、免疫系统、消化系统、血液系统、泌尿系统、内分泌系统与性腺系统的功能变化。应激是机体对多种强烈刺激的一种保护性反应，但在反应失调时，对机体产生不良的影响，包括应激性疾病、心身疾病和心理、精神障碍。

本实验由学生根据课堂所学有关应激的理论知识，结合国内外相关研究，自行设计一个动物实验，使学生在巩固书本知识的同时，进一步开拓思维。在实验设计过程中，应注意思考以下几个问题：

1. 应激源的选择、动物的选择以及如何制备应激的动物模型？

2. 应激时机体的主要表现是什么？

3. 哪些指标可用来判断机体是否出现应激反应及应激反应的程度？

4. 可以应用哪些药物加重或减轻机体的应激性损伤？

（吴　静　门秀丽）

第七章 机能实验学强化训练

习 题 一

一、填空题

1. 机能实验以动物实验为主，根据实验目的不同，可以采取不同的实验方法，主要包括_____和_____两种。

2. 实验报告的核心是_____。

3. 实验结果的表达方式，可按不同类型的实验结果选用_____、_____、_____ 3 种表达方式中的一种或几种。

4. 实验讨论部分是实验结果的_____，是实验报告的_____。

5. 在机能实验中最常用的换能器有_____和_____两种。

6. 描记家兔呼吸运动用_____换能器。描记家兔动脉血压用_____换能器。

7. 在 BL - 420 生物机能实验系统中分时复用区包括_____、_____、和_____、_____四个功能区。

8. 在 BL - 420 生物机能实验系统中有_____和_____两种类型的实验标记供选择。

9. BL - 420 生物机能实验系统中调节增益的作用是_____。

10. _____和_____的目的是为了将需要观察的生物机能信号从其他机能信号或噪声信号中分离出来。

11. 家兔全身麻醉过程中，麻醉的深浅可以根据_____、_____、_____、_____等来判断。

12. 家兔颈部动脉鞘中包含三根神经，其中最粗的是_____，最细的是_____。

13. 分离血管神经的分离原则是：先_____后_____，先_____后_____。

14. 常用的家兔捉拿方法为：用右手抓住_____将其提起，然后用左手_____，使兔身的重量大部分落于左手上。

二、单项选择题

1. 实验报告的主体是指
   A. 实验结论　　　　　　B. 实验结果
   C. 实验步骤　　　　　　D. 实验讨论

2. 从实验结果中归纳出一般的概括性判断是
   A. 实验结论　　　　　　B. 实验讨论
   C. 实验原理　　　　　　D. 实验目的

3. 当血压波形振幅较大或较小时，可调节哪个按钮
   A. 时间常数　　　　　　B. 高频滤波
   C. 扫描速度　　　　　　D. 增益

4. 在使用 BL - 420 生物机能实验系统进行实验过程中，要不断观察生物信号测量的数

据，通常需用鼠标单击分时复用区中的哪个按钮

A. 通用信息显示区

B. 控制参数调节区

C. 显示参数调节区

D. 标尺调节区

5. 在 BL－420 生物机能实验系统中，下列哪个图标表示为记录存盘状态

A. ▶　　　　　　　　B. ●

C. ■　　　　　　　　D. ❚❚

6. 波形较宽或较窄时，可调节哪个按钮

A. 时间常数　　　　　B. 滤波

C. 扫描速度　　　　　D. 增益

7. 家兔实验中分离颈部神经血管的原则是

A. 先神经后血管，先细后粗

B. 先血管后神经，先细后粗

C. 先血管后神经，先粗后细

D. 先神经后血管，先粗后细

8. 给家兔进行全身麻醉时，乌拉坦用量为

A. 1 g/kg　　　　　　B. 2 g/kg

C. 4 ml/kg　　　　　D. 5 ml/kg

9. 家兔颈部手术时，打开动脉鞘时，可见最细的神经是

A. 迷走神经　　　　　B. 交感神经

C. 升压神经　　　　　D. 减压神经

10. 在机能学实验中，颈总动脉插管是一项常用的实验技术，将分离好的颈总动脉尽量靠_____心端用线结扎，在_____心端用动脉夹夹闭血管。

A. 近；远　　　　　　B. 远；近

C. 远；远　　　　　　D. 近；近

11. 手术镊的正确握持方法是

A. 持镊时，用拇指对食指

B. 持镊时，用拇指对食指和中指

C. 持镊时，用拇指对食指、中指和无名指

D. 握在掌心，利于镊子稳定

12. 下列关于眼科剪叙述正确的是

A. 常用来剪包膜、神经

B. 常用来剪皮肤、肌肉

C. 常用来剪神经、肌肉

D. 常用来剪肌肉、骨骼

三、多项选择题

1. 实验报告包括以下哪些内容

A. 实验目的和原理

B. 实验动物、器材和试剂

C. 实验方法和步骤

D. 实验结果和分析

2. 实验报告的结论

A. 是从结果和讨论中归纳出来的

B. 反映学生对实验结果的理论认识

C. 以实验结果为依据

D. 是实验报告的核心

3. 讨论的内容包括

A. 以实验结果为论据，论证实验目的

B. 根据已知的理论知识对结果进行解释和分析

C. 分析实验中出现的非预期的结果

D. 实验公式的推导计算

4. 实验结果是

A. 指实验材料经实验过程加工处理后得到的结果

B. 实验报告的概括性判断

C. 实验报告的核心

D. 实验报告的主体

5. 在使用 BL－420 生物机能实验系统时，下列哪些有消除干扰的作用

A. 增益　　　　　　　B. 滤波

C. 时间常数　　　　　D. 50 Hz 滤波

6. 在机能实验中使用张力换能器的实验有哪些

A. 呼吸运动调节

B. 组胺及抗组胺药物对离体回肠作用

C. 刺激强度和刺激频率对骨骼肌收缩影响

D. 期前收缩及代偿间歇

7. 关于手术器械的使用，错误的是

A. 手术剪适用于剪神经、血管、骨头等组织

B. 止血钳用来夹闭出血点，分离组织等，不宜用其夹持血管、脏器及脆弱的组织

C. 使用持针器时，用其尖端夹住缝合针近尾端 1/3 处

D. 眼科剪常用来剪包膜、皮肤、肌肉等组织，禁用剪骨骼

8. 手术剪适用于剪以下哪种组织

A. 神经　　　　　　　B. 血管

C. 脂肪　　　　　　　D. 骨组织

9. 关于静脉麻醉下列说法正确的是

A. 静脉注射麻醉作用发生快，没有明显的兴奋期，几乎立即生效

B. 静脉麻醉常缓慢注射麻醉药，若肌肉松弛，呼吸减慢，角膜反射消失，表示麻醉药已足量

C. 麻醉药的用量与动物体重成正比，麻醉药浓度越高麻醉效果越好

D. 静脉注射麻醉时，随时观察动物反应，给药速度应缓慢

10. 全身麻醉的给药途径有

A. 静脉注射　　　　　B. 腹腔注射

C. 皮下浸润　　　　　D. 吸入

四、判断题

（　　）1. 实验结论就是简单地把实验结果总结到一起。

（　　）2. 从实验结果中归纳出一般的概括性判断是实验结论。

（　　）3. 滤波是指低通滤波或高频滤波，即衰减信号中的高频成分，而让低频成分全部通过。

（　　）4. 心血管运动的神经-体液调节实验中，使用 BL－420 生物机能实验系统描记血压时用的换能器为张力换能器。

（　　）5. BL－420 生物机能实验系统进入实验状态的方式（即输入方式）有从实验项目进入和从输入信号进入（输入信号—几通道—张力）两种。

（　　）6. 捉拿家兔时，要右手抓耳朵，左手托住家兔的臀部，大部分重量落于左手上。

（　　）7. 止血钳用来夹闭出血点，分离组织等，不宜用其夹持血管、脏器及脆弱的组织。

（　　）8. 静脉麻醉时麻醉药用量与动物体重成正比，麻醉药浓度越高麻醉效果越好。

（　　）9. 家兔耳缘静脉注射时应选择近耳根部较粗的部位进针。

（　　）10. 静脉注射时，将有无回血作为判断静脉注射是否准确的唯一标准。

（　　）11. 眼科剪常用来剪包膜、神经、血管组织，禁用剪毛、皮肤、肌肉、骨骼等组织。

五、简答题

1. 使用 BL－420 生物机能实验系统监测家兔心电图时，心电图的干扰较大，可能原因有哪些？如何解决？

2. 家兔耳缘静脉注射氨基甲酸乙酯溶液麻醉过程中，应注意观察动物哪些特征改变？

3. 家兔实验手术操作过程中如果出现出血，应如何处理？

习题一参考答案

一、填空题

1. 急性实验　慢性实验
2. 实验结果
3. 叙述式　表格式　简图式
4. 逻辑延伸　主体
5. 张力换能器　压力换能器
6. 张力　压力
7. 控制参数调节区　显示参数调节区　通用信息显示区　专用信息显示区
8. 通用标记　特殊标记
9. 调节波形的大小
10. 滤波　时间常数
11. 角膜反射　肌张力　对疼痛刺激的反应　呼吸
12. 迷走神经　减压神经
13. 神经　血管　细　粗
14. 颈背部的被毛与皮　托住其臀部

二、单项选择题

1. D　2. A　3. D　4. A　5. B　6. C　7. A　8. A　9. D　10. B　11. B　12. A

三、多项选择题

1. ABCD　2. ABC　3. ABC　4. AC　5. BCD　6. ABCD　7. AD　8. ABC
9. ABD　10. ABD

四、判断题

1. ×　2. √　3. √　4. ×　5. √　6. ×　7. √　8. ×　9. ×　10. ×　11. √

五、简答题

1. 答：使用 BL-420 生物机能实验系统实验时，心电图的干扰较大可能原因：（1）心电输入线接触不良。（2）心电输入线接地不好。（3）心电输入线没有充分与动物肢体接触。（4）动物肌电或其他干扰信号的影响。解决方法：（1）检查心电输入线是否接触良好。（2）检查计算机接地是否良好。（3）将引导插针插入到动物肢体的皮毛下面。（4）等动物安静一段时间再观察其心电波形。（5）调节 "T"、"F" 按钮。

2. 答：麻醉过程中，麻醉的深浅可依据角膜反射、肌张力、对疼痛刺激的反应、呼吸判断。若角膜反射迟钝或消失、肌肉松弛、呼吸减慢、痛反应消失，表明药物已足量。

3. 答：手术操作过程中如果出现出血，应及时处理，不要惊慌。

（1）少量出血可用盐水纱布压迫出血部位直至出血停止，如静脉注射穿刺点出血或切皮时少量出血时，可采用此法。（2）出血量较大时，应迅速清理手术野，找到出血点；用止血钳将出血点夹闭或用手术线将出血点结扎。

（王银环　杨秀红）

习 题 二

一、填空题

1. 调节呼吸运动的外周化学感受器是_____和_____。

2. 当动脉血液中 PO_2_____，PCO_2_____时，可引起呼吸运动加强。

3. 由家兔耳缘静脉注射乳酸后，主要通过刺激_____感受器，使呼吸加深加快。

4. 剪断家兔两侧迷走神经后，呼吸变得_____，吸气过程_____，机制是_____。

5. 当动脉血 PCO_2 突然增大时，_____感受器最先引起快速呼吸反应。动脉血 PCO_2 突然增大引起的呼吸变化中起主要作用的是_____感受器。

6. 支配心脏的传出神经为_____和_____。

7. 兔颈总动脉血压曲线一级波是由于_____形成。

8. 压力感受性反射是通过对_____和_____压力感受器的刺激而引起的。

9. 在心血管运动神经体液调节实验中，向心方向牵拉颈总动脉头端时，血压_____。

10. 正常的血压曲线的三级波型中，一级波代表_____，二级波代表_____，三级波是由于_____所致。

11. 向家兔静脉内快速注射 20％ 的葡萄糖，此时家兔尿量_____，属于_____利尿。

12. 给家兔静脉注射大量生理盐水引起尿量_____，主要原因是_____和_____。

13. 肾小球滤过的动力是肾小球有效滤过压，是_____、_____和_____三者的代数和。

二、单项选择题

1. 在动物实验中，人为地在气管插管一端接上 40 cm 长的橡皮管以增加无效腔，将会出现哪种情况
   A. 呼吸变快、变浅
   B. 呼吸加深、加快
   C. 呼吸变浅、变慢
   D. 窒息死亡

2. 切断兔双侧迷走神经后，呼吸的改变是
   A. 呼吸幅度减小
   B. 吸气相延长

C. 呼吸频率加快

D. 血液 CO_2 张力暂时升高

3. 下列关于肺牵张反射的叙述哪项是正确的

A. 平静呼吸时参与人的呼吸调节

B. 肺牵张反射即肺扩张反射

C. 肺牵张感受器位于肺泡壁

D. 肺扩张反射的作用在于加速吸气向呼气的转换

4. 下列关于无效腔的叙述哪项是不正确的

A. 肺泡无效腔是由于肺内血流分布不均造成

B. 健康人平卧时的生理无效腔大于解剖无效腔

C. 肺泡通气量等于（潮气量－无效腔气量）×呼吸频率

D. 生理无效腔等于解剖无效腔与肺泡无效腔之和

5. CO_2 增强呼吸运动主要是通过刺激哪种感受器

A. 中枢化学感受器

B. 压力感受器

C. 牵张感受器

D. 外周化学感受器

6. 延髓中枢化学感受器的生理刺激是

A. 动脉血中 CO_2 浓度升高

B. 脑脊液中 CO_2 浓度升高

C. 血液中〔H^+〕升高

D. 脑脊液中〔H^+〕升高

7. 分别刺激下列神经后会引起动脉血压升高的是

A. 交感神经 　　　B. 减压神经

C. 迷走神经 　　　D. 副神经

8. 在动物实验中，当夹闭家兔右侧颈总脉时

A. 血压升高

B. 心率减慢

C. 窦神经传入冲动增加

D. 血管运动中枢活动减弱

9. 心血管运动调节实验中，夹闭右侧兔颈总动脉引起血压升高的主要原因是

A. 颈动脉窦受到牵拉刺激

B. 颈动脉窦受到缺氧刺激

C. 颈动脉窦感受到的刺激减弱，窦神经传入冲动减少

D. 颈动脉窦感受到的刺激减弱，窦神经传入冲动增多

10. 关于压力感受性反射，下列哪一项是错误的

A. 在平时安静状态下不起作用

B. 也称为减压反射

C. 是一种负反馈调节机制

D. 对搏动性的血压改变更加敏感

11. 颈动脉窦和主动脉弓压力感受器的适宜刺激是

A. 颈动脉窦内血压

B. 机体血压

C. 血管壁的被动扩张

D. 主动脉弓内血压

12. 兔主动脉弓压力感受器的传入神经是

A. 迷走神经 　　　B. 窦神经

C. 减压神经 　　　D. 舌咽神经

13. 刺激家兔减压神经头端时血压下降，而刺激心端血压不变，这一现象说明

A. 减压神经传入冲动增多

B. 减压神经为混合神经

C. 减压神经为传出神经

D. 减压神经为传入神经

14. 抗利尿激素分泌的有效刺激是血浆晶体渗透压的增高和＿＿＿＿＿的减少

A. 循环血量 　　　B. 胶体渗透压

C. 肾小管重吸收 　　D. 集合管重吸收

15. 在影响尿生成因素实验中用到的指示剂为

A. 酚红 　　　　　B. 氢氧化钠

C. 龙胆紫 　　　　D. 苦味酸

16. 速尿产生利尿作用的部位是

A. 近曲小管 　　　B. 髓袢降支

C. 髓袢升支 　　　D. 远曲小管

17. 下列原因中直接引起渗透性利尿是

A. 肾小球滤过率增加

B. 血浆晶体渗透压升高

C. 小管液中溶质浓度升高

D. 远曲小管和集合管对水的通透性降低

18. 抗利尿激素的作用是

A. 促进远曲小管和集合管对水的重吸收

B. 促进远曲小管和集合管保 Na^+ 排 K^+

C. 减少内髓部集合管对尿素的通透

D. 促进远曲小管和髓袢对水的重吸收

19. 下列可导致肾小球滤过率降低的是

A. 注射大量高渗葡萄糖液

B. 注射去甲肾上腺素

C. 快速静脉滴注生理盐水

D. 注射抗利尿激素

20. 下列情况中可使肾小球滤过率增加的是

A. 快速输入生理盐水

B. 剧烈运动

C. 大量出汗

D. 静脉输入白蛋白

21. 下列实验结果中，错误的是

A. 静脉注射 10^{-4} mol/L 去甲肾上腺素 0.5 ml，尿量增加

B. 电刺激迷走神经外周端，尿量减少

C. 静注 20% 葡萄糖 5 ml，尿量增加

D. 静脉注射垂体后叶素 2 单位，尿量减少

三、多项选择题

1. CO_2 对呼吸的调节是通过

A. 直接刺激延髓呼吸中枢

B. 加强肺牵张反射

C. 刺激颈动脉体和主动脉体化学感受器

D. 刺激延髓中枢化学感受器

2. 下列干预因素中，可使呼吸加深加快的有哪些

A. 增加吸入气中 CO_2 浓度

B. 增大无效腔

C. 耳缘静脉注射 3% 乳酸溶液

D. 剪断双侧迷走神经

3. 实验中家兔气管插管连接 40 cm 长橡胶管时，呼吸加深加快主要原因是

A. 本体感受性反射减弱

B. 呼吸肌本体感受性反射增强

C. 动脉血 PCO_2 升高

D. 动脉血 PO_2 降低

4. 关于肺牵张反射的叙述，正确的是

A. 感受器位于肺泡壁上

B. 传入神经是迷走神经

C. 使呼气转为吸气

D. 肺充气或扩张时抑制吸气

5. 下列选项中能引起血压升高的是

A. 交感神经兴奋

B. 静脉注射肾上腺素

C. 静脉注射去甲肾上腺素

D. 电刺激迷走神经

6. 一般情况下判断动静脉血管的标准有

A. 动脉血管的颜色较为鲜红或淡红色

B. 静脉血管的颜色为深红或紫红色

C. 动脉血管看似刚劲，有明显的搏动现象

D. 静脉血管看似单薄、无搏动感

7. 下列实验操作中能使血压降低的是

A. 电刺激迷走神经

B. 电刺激减压神经头端

C. 夹闭右侧颈总动脉

D. 向心方向牵拉颈总动脉头端

8. 导致肾小球有效滤过压增高的因素是

A. 血浆胶体渗透压增高

B. 肾小球毛细血管静水压升高

C. 血浆胶体渗透压降低

D. 血浆晶体渗透压降低

9. 影响肾小管重吸收和分泌的因素包括

A. 静脉注入高渗葡萄糖

B. 醛固酮

C. 交感神经系统

D. 抗利尿激素

10. 下列哪种情况使肾小球滤过率下降

A. 肾小球毛细血管血压升高

B. 肾小球血浆流量减少

C. 肾小球滤过面积减少

D. 囊内压升高

11. 以下哪些属于渗透性利尿

A. 大量饮水使尿量增多

B. 糖尿病患者的多尿

C. 静滴 20％甘露醇

D. 静滴 5％葡萄糖 500 ml

12. 影响尿生成因素的实验结果中，错误的是

A. 静注大量生理盐水，尿量增加

B. 静注 10^{-4} mol/L 去甲肾上腺素 0.5 ml，

尿量增加

C. 静注速尿，尿量增加

D. 静注垂体后叶素后，尿量增加

13. 尿生成影响因素实验中，开始实验尚未给药时，尿量很少或无尿，可能原因有

A. 实验前给兔饲喂菜叶少，机体缺水

B. 兔本身机能状态欠佳

C. 输尿管或插管内有血凝块堵塞

D. 腹部切口暴露太大或手术创伤等致使血压下降，并反射性引起 ADH 分泌

四、判断题

( ) 1. 呼吸的无效腔越大，则肺泡通气量越小。

( ) 2. 在呼吸调节实验中，每次观察完一个实验项目后，可立即进行下一个实验项目。

( ) 3. 给家兔耳缘静脉注射 3％乳酸溶液时，总量一般不超过 2 ml。

( ) 4. CO_2 增强呼吸运动主要是通过刺激外周化学感受器发挥作用。

( ) 5. 实验中可挡住气管插管另一侧支的一半，以增大气道阻力。

( ) 6. 进行血压测量时，应保持压力换能器与动物心脏呈同一水平状态，以保证测量血压数据的准确性。

( ) 7. 家兔减压神经为主动脉弓压力感受器的传入神经，剪断减压神经刺激向心端血压基本不变。

( ) 8. 因为去甲肾上腺素有升高血压的作用，所以注射时要缓慢，以免血压升高过快。

( ) 9. 当尿中出现葡萄糖时，尿中糖的浓度为肾糖阈。

( ) 10. 大量饮清水后尿量增多的主要原因为血浆胶体渗透压降低。

( ) 11. 进行影响尿生成的因素实验时，要注意给药顺序，按照尿量增多、减少交替的顺序进行。

( ) 12. 决定尿量多少的主要环节是肾小球滤过率，而不是肾小管与集合管对水的重吸收。

( ) 13. 肾小管液中的葡萄糖主要在远曲小管被全部重吸收。

五、简答题

1. 呼吸运动调节实验中，增加无效腔气量如何操作？呼吸有何改变？机制是什么？

2. 在心血管运动的神经体液调节实验中，短时夹闭右侧颈总动脉对全身血压有何影响？为什么？

3. 尿生成影响因素实验中，静脉注射垂体后叶素后尿量如何改变？简述其机制。

习题二参考答案

一、填空题

1. 颈动脉体　主动脉体
2. 降低　升高
3. 外周化学
4. 深而慢　延长　阻断迷走神经参与的肺牵张反射通路
5. 外周化学　中枢化学
6. 心交感神经　心迷走神经
7. 心脏搏动
8. 颈动脉窦　主动脉弓
9. 降低
10. 心搏波　呼吸波　血管紧张性周期性变化
11. 增加　渗透性
12. 增加　血浆胶体渗透压降低　肾血流量增加
13. 肾小球毛细血管静水压　肾小囊内压　血浆胶体渗透压

二、单项选择题

1. B　2. B　3. D　4. B　5. A　6. D　7. A　8. A　9. C　10. A　11. C　12. C　13. D　14. A　15. A　16. C　17. C　18. A　19. B　20. A　21. A

三、多项选择题

1. CD　2. ABC　3. CD　4. BCD　5. ABC　6. ABCD　7. ABD　8. BC　9. ABCD　10. BCD　11. BC　12. BD　13. ABCD

四、判断题

1. √　2. ×　3. √　4. ×　5. √　6. √　7. √　8. ×　9. ×　10. ×　11. √　12. ×　13. ×

五、简答题

1. 答：（1）将长的胶管连于气管插管的侧管上以增加无效腔。（2）可以看到呼吸加深加快。（3）机制：将长的胶管连于气管插管的侧管上，可增大解剖无效腔，使肺泡通气量减少，PO_2↓（起主要作用），PCO_2↑，从而刺激颈动脉体和主动脉体化学感受器，冲动分别经窦神经和迷走神经传入延髓，反射性地引起呼吸加深加快。

2. 答：（1）血压一过性升高后恢复正常水平。（2）机制：夹闭一侧颈总动脉后，局部压力减小，窦内压下降，位于颈部的压力感受器——颈动脉窦压力感受器感受机械牵张刺激减弱，经窦神经上传冲动减少，反射性的使迷走紧张减弱，交感紧张加强，于是心率加快，心输出量增加，外周血管阻力增高，血压升高。

3. 答：尿量减少。

机制：垂体后叶素中影响尿量变化的是抗利尿激素（ADH），ADH 主要通过以下途径使尿量减少。（1）提高远曲小管和集合管上皮细胞对水的通透性，增加水的重吸收，使尿液浓缩，尿量减少。（2）增加髓袢升支粗段对 NaCl 的主动重吸收和内髓部集合管对尿素的通透性，从而增加髓质组织间液的溶质浓度，提高髓质组织间液的渗透压，有利于水的重吸收，尿量减少。（3）垂体后叶素用量较大时，还可使肾血管收缩，肾血流量减少，肾小球毛细血管静水压降低，肾小球有效滤过压下降，滤过减少，尿量减少。

（王银环　杨秀红）

习 题 三

一、填空题

1. 如果后一刺激引起的收缩落于前一刺激引起的收缩过程的舒张期内，在描记曲线上形成锯齿形，此种收缩形式称为_____。

2. 如果后一刺激引起的收缩落于前一刺激引起的收缩过程的收缩期内，在描记曲线上形成平滑、持续的收缩曲线，此种收缩形式称为_____。

3. 刺激强度逐步增大时，肌肉收缩反应也相应增大，当肌肉收缩不再随刺激强度增加而增大时，此时的收缩即为_____。

4. 能引起细胞产生动作电位的最小的刺激强度，称为_____。

5. 相当于阈强度的刺激称为_____。

6. 骨骼肌受到刺激后发生收缩反应的过程包括_____、_____和_____。

7. 在心室舒张中、晚期给予心室一次适宜的刺激，可引起一次比正常节律早的收缩，称为_____。

8. 在体蛙心实验常用的营养液是_____，蛙心的正常起搏点是_____。

9. 在一次期前收缩之后，往往有一段较长的心室舒张期，称为_____。

10. 与骨骼肌相比，心肌兴奋性周期性变化的特点在于其_____。

二、单项选择题

1. 机能学实验中处死蟾蜍的方法一般采用
   A. 腹腔注射　　　B. 皮下注射
   C. 破坏脑和脊髓　D. 断头

2. 蟾蜍的坐骨神经位于_____之间
   A. 股二头肌和半膜肌
   B. 大内直肌和大收肌

133

C. 缝匠肌和外侧肌膜

D. 半膜肌和缝匠肌

3. 判断组织兴奋性高低常用的指标是

   A. 阈电位

   B. 刺激频率

   C. 阈强度

   D. 刺激强度的变化率

4. 在正常人体内，骨骼肌收缩属于

   A. 不完全强直收缩

   B. 强直收缩和单收缩

   C. 强直收缩

   D. 单收缩

5. 心室期前收缩之后出现代偿间歇的原因是

   A. 来自窦房结的兴奋传导速度大大减慢

   B. 窦房结的节律兴奋少发放一次

   C. 窦性期前兴奋的有效不应期特别长

   D. 窦房结发出的兴奋落在期前兴奋的有效不应期中

6. 在有效不应期，下列说法正确的是

   A. 无论多么强的刺激都不能引起任何反应

   B. 需要阈上刺激才能产生动作电位

C. 不能产生动作电位

D. 阈下刺激也可以诱发动作电位

7. 在绝对不应期，下列说法正确的是

   A. 足够强的刺激可引起局部去极化反应

   B. 需要阈上刺激才能诱发动作电位

   C. 不能产生动作电位

   D. 阈下刺激可以诱发去极化反应

8. 在相对不应期，下列说法正确的是

   A. 无论多么强的刺激都不能引起反应

   B. 需要阈上刺激才能发生动作电位

   C. 不能产生动作电位

   D. 阈下刺激也可以诱发动作电位

9. 在超常期，下列说法正确的是

   A. 无论多么强的刺激都不能引起反应

   B. 只有阈上刺激才能发生反应

   C. 不能产生动作电位

   D. 阈下刺激也可诱发动作电位

10. 在以下何时给予心室一个额外刺激不引起期前收缩

    A. 心室收缩期　　B. 心室舒张中期

    C. 心室舒张晚期　D. 有效不应期后

三、多项选择题

1. 一份完整的蛙坐骨神经-腓肠肌标本包括

   A. 下 2/3 股骨　　　　B. 膝关节

   C. 坐骨神经　　　　　D. 腓肠肌

2. 下列说法正确的是

   A. 任意刺激强度下给予神经肌肉标本一单独或一连串的电刺激，可使肌肉出现不同形式的收缩

   B. 在动物实验中给予肌肉一连串电刺激使其发生收缩，后一刺激引起的肌肉收缩落在前一刺激引起肌肉收缩的舒张期时，可出现完全强直收缩

   C. 给予肌肉一连串电刺激使其发生收缩，刺激的时间间隔大于一个单收缩的收缩期和舒张期之和，可产生一连串的单收缩

D. 给予肌肉一连串电刺激使其发生收缩，后一刺激引起的肌肉收缩落在前一刺激引起肌肉收缩的舒张期时，可出现不完全强直收缩

3. 在骨骼肌的单复合收缩实验中，若给予刺激后未观察到收缩曲线，可能的原因有

   A. 标本制备过程中神经受损

   B. 标本干燥

   C. 刺激强度过小

   D. 神经与刺激电极接触不良

4. 下列关于骨骼肌动作电位与收缩的关系叙述正确的是

   A. 肌肉的不完全强直收缩所描记到的波形为锯齿形

   B. 单收缩和完全强直收缩所描记到的波

形为直线

C. 肌细胞的动作电位总是在机械收缩之前出现

D. 骨骼肌前一次刺激引起的收缩还未完全舒张时，新的阈上刺激到达肌肉，对肌肉无任何作用

5. 下列说法正确的是

A. 在心室舒张中、晚期内给予心室一次适宜刺激，可引起一次期前收缩

B. 在心肌兴奋的绝对不应期内，任何强大的刺激均不能引起心肌收缩

C. 在心肌兴奋的相对不应期内，任何强大的刺激均不能引起心肌收缩

D. 心肌不会发生强直收缩

6. 期前收缩后出现代偿间歇是由于

A. 窦房结的自律性降低

B. 期前收缩的舒张期延长

C. 窦性冲动落在期前收缩的收缩期或舒张早期

D. 窦性心率较快，下一次窦房结的兴奋正好落在期前兴奋的有效不应期内

7. 在期前收缩和代偿间歇实验中，为保证实验的准确性，应该注意

A. 破坏蟾蜍的脑和脊髓要完全

B. 不能完全破坏蟾蜍的脑和脊髓，以保证心肌具有足够的兴奋性

C. 蛙心夹与张力换能器间的连线应有一定的紧张度

D. 注意滴加林格液，以保持蛙心适宜的环境

8. 在两栖类实验过程中要注意滴加林格液，主要原因是

A. 林格液中含有组织正常生命活动必需的营养物质和电解质

B. 林格液渗透压和酸碱度与动物体液相似

C. 林格液可以增加组织的兴奋性

D. 林格液就是生理盐水

9. 心肌细胞动作电位平台期的长短决定了

A. 有效不应期的长短

B. 收缩期的长短

C. 超常期的长短

D. 整个动作电位时程的长短

10. 影响心肌细胞兴奋性的因素有

A. 阈电位水平　　　　B. 静息电位水平

C. 0 期去极速度　　　D. 4 期去极速度

四、判断题

（　）1. 两栖类动物实验中常用到的溶液是生理盐水。

（　）2. 刺激坐骨神经-腓肠肌标本时要将刺激强度调到最大，以便更好地观察实验现象。

（　）3. 只要给予神经肌肉标本一单独或一连串的电刺激，就可使肌肉出现不同的收缩形式。

（　）4. 给予肌肉一连串电刺激使其发生收缩时，如果刺激的时间间隔大于一个单收缩的收缩期和舒张期之和，可产生一连串的单收缩。

（　）5. 阈下刺激可引起可兴奋细胞产生局部反应，局部反应具有"全或无"的特性。

（　）6. 骨骼肌的收缩过程需要消耗 ATP，舒张过程是一种弹性复原，无需消耗 ATP。

（　）7. 阈下刺激不会引起心脏产生任何生理反应。

（　）8. 蛙心的正常起搏点是窦房结。

（　）9. 期前收缩之后不一定会出现代偿间歇。

（　）10. 心肌跟骨骼肌一样，受到连续的阈上刺激可引起强直收缩。

（　）11. 心肌动作电位的时程长于骨骼肌的动作电位时程。

（　）12. 在心肌有效不应期内，无论给予多强的刺激也不会产生膜的任何程度的去极化。

（　）13. 在相对不应期内，无论多强的刺激也不会引起细胞发生兴奋。

五、简答题

1. 画图并说明何谓不完全强直收缩和完全强直收缩？阐述其发生的原理。

2. 为什么在一定范围内刺激强度增大肌肉收缩的幅度也增大？

3. 在期前收缩之后，为什么会出现代偿间歇？

4. 心率过快或过缓时，期前收缩后是否会出现代偿间歇？为什么？

习题三参考答案

一、填空题

1. 不完全强直收缩

2. 完全强直收缩

3. 最大收缩

4. 阈强度

5. 阈刺激

6. 潜伏期　收缩期　舒张期

7. 期前收缩

8. 林格液　静脉窦

9. 代偿间歇

10. 有效不应期特别长

二、单项选择题

1. C　2. A　3. C　4. C　5. D　6. C　7. C　8. B　9. D　10. A

三、多项选择题

1. ABCD　2. CD　3. ABCD　4. AC　5. ABD　6. CD　7. ACD　8. AB　9. AD　10. AB

四、判断题

1. ×　2. ×　3. ×　4. √　5. ×　6. ×　7. ×　8. ×　9. √　10. ×　11. √　12. ×　13. ×

五、简答题

1. 答：当骨骼肌受到频率较高的连续刺激时，可出现收缩过程的总和，即为强直收缩。

（1）如果刺激频率相对较低，总和过程发生于前一次收缩过程的舒张期，将出现不完全强直收缩，表现为锯齿状的收缩曲线（见图7-1）。（2）如果刺激频率相对较高，总和过程发生于前一次收缩过程的收缩期，将出现完全强直收缩，表现为平滑、持续的收缩曲线（见图7-2）。

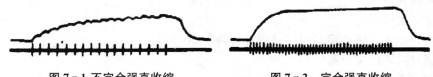

图7-1 不完全强直收缩　　　图7-2 完全强直收缩

原理：骨骼肌动作电位持续时间短，仅2～4 ms，绝对不应期特别短，而收缩过程可达几十甚至几百毫秒，因而骨骼肌有可能在机械收缩过程中接受新的刺激并发生新的兴奋和收缩。

2. 答：单根神经纤维或肌纤维对刺激的反应是"全或无"式的，但在神经肌肉标本中，则表现为一定范围内肌肉收缩的幅度同刺激神经的强度成正比。因为坐骨神经干中含有数十万条粗细不等的神经纤维，其兴奋性不相同。弱刺激只能使其中少量兴奋性高的神经纤维先兴奋，并引起它所支配的少量肌纤维收缩。随着刺激强度增大，发生兴奋的神经纤维数目增多，结果肌肉收缩幅度随刺激强度的增加而增强。当刺激达到一定程度，神经干中全部神经纤维均兴奋，其所支配的全部肌纤维也都发生兴奋和收缩，从而引起肌肉的最大收缩。此后，若再增加刺激强度，肌肉收缩幅度将不再增加。

3. 答：正常心脏按窦房结的节律有规律地收缩和舒张，但若在心室兴奋的有效不应期之后，下一次窦房结兴奋到达前，心肌受到了人工的刺激或窦房结之外的病理性刺激，心室也可产生一次正常节律以外的兴奋和收缩，称为期前收缩（也称早搏）。而期前兴奋也有其自身的有效不应期，当紧接在期前收缩后的又一次正常的窦房结兴奋传到心室时，若恰好落在期前兴奋的有效不应期之内，则不能引起心室产生新的兴奋和收缩，必须要等到下次窦房结的兴奋传来时，才能引起心室收缩。这样，在一次期前收缩之后，往往有一段较长的心室舒张期，称为代偿间歇。

4. 答：（1）如果心率过快，快到本身的节律就已经使心肌产生不完全强直收缩的程度，心肌本身就没有充分地舒张，舒张中、晚期很短，这时候额外的刺激就可能没有机会落在舒张中、晚期，而只能落在心肌收缩的收缩期和舒张早期（有效不应期），因此就不会产生期前收缩和代偿间歇。（2）如果心率太慢，在舒张中、晚期给予额外刺激，可以产生期前收缩。但是心率慢到后一次窦性节律落在了期前兴奋的有效不应期之后（例如落在相对不应期、超常期，甚至已经完全恢复到静息期），这时候就不会产生代偿间歇。

（张　娜　杨秀红）

习 题 四

一、填空题

1. 高钾血症对机体酸碱平衡会产生影响，可诱发_____，尿液呈_____性。

2. 高钾血症可由于_____、_____、_____引起。

3. 高钾血症对心脏损害严重，最终心脏停搏于_____，机制是心肌细胞膜对 K^+ 通透性_____，细胞内 K^+ 外流_____，Ca^{2+} 内流_____，收缩性减弱。

4. 正常血钾浓度为_____。高钾血症是指血清钾浓度高于_____的状态，低钾血症是指血清钾浓度低于_____的状态。

5. 实验中高钾血症的抢救步骤包括立即停止注射 KCl 溶液_____和_____。

6. 高钾血症对机体的主要影响和威胁是_____和_____。

7. 毛细血管中脱氧血红蛋白平均浓度增加到_____以上可使皮肤黏膜呈青紫色。

8. 严重低 O_2 对呼吸中枢有_____的作用。

9. 常用的血氧指标有_____、_____、_____、_____。

10. 低张性缺氧主要特点为_____，从而使_____降低，组织_____。

11. "氨在肝性脑病发生中的作用"实验中，结扎的三个肝叶分别是_____、_____、_____。

12. 氨中毒学说认为肝性脑病的发生是由于肝功能严重受损，_____合成发生障碍而导致_____水平增高，引起脑功能障碍。

13. 肝功能严重障碍者需灌肠时应选用_____性溶液。

14. "氨在肝性脑病发生中的作用"实验中，家兔典型的体征改变是_____，表现为四肢伸直，头尾昂起，脊柱挺硬。

15. 肝性脑病的发生主要是脑组织_____和_____障碍所致。

二、单项选择题

1. 高钾血症时不包括
   A. 心肌传导性下降
   B. 心肌自律性下降
   C. 心律失常
   D. 代谢性碱中毒

2. 高钾血症时，心电图的特点是
   A. T 波高尖，QT 间期缩短
   B. T 波高尖，QT 间期延长
   C. T 波低平，QT 间期缩短
   D. T 波低平，QT 间期延长

3. 临床上引起高钾血症最主要的原因是
   A. 急性酸中毒引起细胞内 K^+ 释放至细胞外液
   B. 缺氧时细胞内 K^+ 释放至细胞外液
   C. 肾排钾减少
   D. 钾摄入过多

4. 严重高钾血症的主要危险是
   A. 引起严重碱中毒

B. 引起肌肉阵挛收缩
C. 引起心跳突然停止
D. 引起麻痹性肠梗阻

5. 下述哪项不是高钾血症的原因
   A. β-肾上腺素受体阻断剂
   B. 胰岛素过量使用
   C. 酸中毒
   D. 急性肾功能衰竭少尿期

6. 缺氧是指
   A. 血液中氧分压下降引起的病理过程
   B. 吸入气中的氧不足引起的病理过程
   C. 对组织供氧不足或组织利用氧障碍引起的病理过程
   D. 血氧含量下降引起的病理过程

7. 有关血氧指标的叙述，下列哪一项不确切
   A. 动脉血氧分压只取决于吸入气中氧分压的高低
   B. 动-静脉血氧含量差可反映内呼吸状况

C. 正常动、静脉血氧含量差是 5 ml/dl

D. 血氧含量是指 100 ml 血液中实际含有氧的毫升数

8. 急性低张性缺氧时机体最重要的代偿反应是

    A. 脑血流量增加

    B. 肺通气量增加

    C. 心肌收缩力增强

    D. 心率加快

9. 动脉血氧分压一般要低于_____，即可刺激外周化学感受器，引起呼吸加深加快

    A. 30 mmHg   B. 40 mmHg

    C. 60 mmHg   D. 80 mmHg

10. 缺氧初期呼吸加深加快，使肺通气量增加。下列对其意义描述错误的是

    A. 降低呼吸面积

    B. 增大呼吸面积

    C. 提高氧的弥散

    D. 增大动脉血氧饱和度

11. 低张性缺氧时细胞发生缺氧的机制是

    A. 毛细血管血量减少

    B. 血氧容量降低

    C. 毛细血管平均氧分压降低

    D. 静脉氧分压降低

12. 促进血氨弥散入肠腔的最主要因素是

    A. 门-体分流   B. 消化道出血

C. 肠内 pH 值上升   D. 肠内 pH 值下降

13. 肝硬化患者血氨升高的原因可以是

    A. 胃肠运动增强   B. 胃肠出血

    C. 脂肪酸摄入减少   D. 糖类摄入减少

14. 肝性脑病的概念是

    A. 肝功能不全所致的精神障碍

    B. 肝功能不全所致的昏迷

    C. 肝功能不全所致的脑部疾病

    D. 肝功能不全所致的精神神经综合征

15. 氨中毒患者脑内能量减少的主要原因是

    A. 三羧酸循环障碍   B. 糖酵解障碍

    C. 脂肪氧化障碍   D. 氨基酸利用障碍

16. 氨对神经细胞膜离子转运的影响是

    A. 细胞内钾增多   B. 细胞外钾增多

    C. 细胞内钠增多   D. 细胞内钠缺乏

17. 胃肠道内妨碍氨吸收的主要因素是

    A. 胆汁分泌减少

    B. 蛋白质摄入减少

    C. 肠道细菌受抑制

    D. 肠道内 pH 小于 5

18. 严重肝病时氨清除不足的主要原因是

    A. 谷氨酰胺合成障碍

    B. 尿素合成障碍

    C. 谷氨酸合成障碍

    D. 丙氨酸合成障碍

三、多项选择题

1. 下列药物中可用以抢救高钾血症的有

    A. 硫酸镁溶液

    B. 10％氯化钙溶液

    C. 4％ NaHCO₃

    D. 葡萄糖-胰岛素溶液

2. 严重高钾血症对骨骼肌的影响是

    A. 肌无力

    B. 处于去极化阻滞状态

    C. 肌麻痹

    D. 静息电位绝对值减小

3. 注射钙剂治疗严重高钾血症的机制是

    A. 使阈电位上移

    B. 使静息电位增大

    C. 恢复心肌的兴奋性

    D. 提高心肌收缩性

4. 导致细胞内钾释放到细胞外液的因素有

    A. 急性酸中毒   B. 血管内溶血

    C. 缺氧   D. 碱中毒

5. 如何减少心电干扰波

    A. 针形电极刺入部位要对称，位于皮下

    B. 导线避免纵横交错

    C. 实验台上的液体要及时排除

D. 导线接地

6. 碳酸氢钠治疗高钾血症的机制是
    A. 促进 K^+ 向细胞内转移
    B. 使 0 期去极化时 Na^+ 内流增加
    C. 缓解酸中毒
    D. 改善心肌传导性

7. 缺氧时循环系统的代偿性反应主要表现在以下几个方面
    A. 心输出量增加
    B. 心率加快
    C. 心收缩力增强
    D. 静脉回流量增加所致

8. 严重缺氧引起心功能障碍的机制是
    A. 心肌 ATP 产生不足
    B. 心肌细胞钙转运异常
    C. 心肌细胞内外钾钠分布异常
    D. 心肌收缩蛋白的破坏

9. 低张性缺氧的血氧指标变化是
    A. PaO_2 降低
    B. 动-静脉血氧含量差减少
    C. 血氧含量减少
    D. 血氧饱和度减少

10. 缺氧瓶内含有钠石灰，其成分是
    A. NaOH
    B. CaO
    C. $NaHCO_3$
    D. $Ca(OH)_2$

11. 在肝性脑病的治疗中，可用_____灌肠

    A. 酸性溶液
    B. 碱性溶液
    C. 乳果糖
    D. 碳酸氢钠

12. 在结扎肝叶时有哪些注意事项
    A. 剪镰状韧带时勿损伤膈肌和血管
    B. 游离肝时动作宜轻以免肝叶破裂出血
    C. 结扎线应扎于肝叶根部
    D. 游离肝胃韧带

13. 血氨升高可影响下列哪些中枢神经递质的含量
    A. 乙酰胆碱
    B. 谷氨酸
    C. 多巴胺
    D. γ-氨基丁酸

14. 肝性脑病的诱因包括
    A. 碱中毒
    B. 消化道出血
    C. 高蛋白饮食
    D. 感染

15. 血 NH_3 升高减少脑 ATP 生成可能通过
    A. 乙酰辅酶 A 生成减少
    B. 大量消耗 NADH
    C. 减少参与三羧酸循环的 α-酮戊二酸
    D. 抑制丙酮酸脱羧酶的活性

16. 肝性脑病时血氨升高的主要原因
    A. 肠道细菌繁殖，分解蛋白质和尿素产氨增多
    B. 肠内氨经肝内、外侧支循环直接进入体循环
    C. 肠内酸透析使氨吸收增多
    D. 肝合成尿素减少

四、判断题

( ) 1. 家兔最后出现室颤时，开胸看到心脏停搏在收缩期。

( ) 2. 体内钾总量减少时，仍可能发生高血钾。

( ) 3. 引起高钾血症的主要原因是代谢性酸中毒。

( ) 4. 家兔发绀表现可通过口唇及动脉插管血液颜色观察。

( ) 5. 低张性缺氧时弥散入组织细胞的氧减少，主要是由于弥散的速度降低引起的。

( ) 6. 氨在肠道被吸收的形式是 NH_4^+。

( ) 7. "氨在肝性脑病发生中的作用"实验，麻醉方法是局部浸润麻醉，所用麻醉剂为普鲁卡因。

( ) 8. 氨在脑内可使谷氨酸和乙酰胆碱生成增多而导致昏迷。

( ) 9. 单纯经十二指肠灌入复方氯化铵溶液不易导致肝性脑病，因为氨可被肝解毒和清除。

（　）10. 辨别家兔肝右中叶的解剖标志是胆囊。

五、简答题

1. 给家兔静脉注射氯化钾后，心电图有哪些改变？阐述其发生的机制。
2. 高钾血症对心肌的生理特性有哪些影响？
3. 发生缺氧后，家兔呼吸有何变化？其发生机制是什么？
4. 简述肝性脑病动物模型的复制方法以及肝性脑病时家兔的表现。
5. 在"氨在肝性脑病发生中的作用"实验中采用哪种麻醉方式？为什么？

习题四参考答案

一、填空题

1. 代谢性酸中毒　碱
2. 钾摄入过多　排出受阻　跨细胞分布异常
3. 舒张期　增高　增加　减少
4. 3.5～5.5 mmol/L　5 mmol/L　3.5 mmol/L
5. $NaHCO_3$快速注射　按摩心脏
6. 各种心律失常　肌无力
7. 5 g/dl
8. 直接抑制
9. 血氧分压　血氧容量　血氧含量　血氧饱和度
10. 动脉血氧分压下降　动脉血氧含量　供氧不足
11. 左中叶　左外叶　右中叶
12. 尿素　血氨
13. 酸
14. 角弓反张
15. 代谢　功能

二、单项选择题

1. D　2. A　3. C　4. C　5. B　6. C　7. A　8. B　9. C　10. A　11. C　12. D　13. B　14. D　15. A　16. B　17. D　18. B

三、多项选择题

1. BCD　2. ABCD　3. ACD　4. ABC　5. ABCD　6. ABCD　7. ABCD　8. ABD　9. ABCD　10. AB　11. AC　12. ABCD　13. ABD　14. ABCD　15. ABCD　16. ABD

四、判断题

1. ×　2. √　3. ×　4. √　5. √　6. ×　7. √　8. ×　9. √　10. √

五、简答题

1. 答：由于传导性降低，心电图上显示 P 波压低、增宽或消失；代表房室传导 PR 间期延长，相当于心室内传导的 QRS 波增宽；相当于心室去极化的 R 波降低。高钾血症时心肌细胞膜的钾通透性明显增高，故钾外流加速，复极化（3 期）加速。因此，动作电位时间和有效不应期均缩短，心电图上显示 T 波狭窄高耸，相当于心室动作电位时间的 QT 间期缩短。

2. 答：（1）对心肌兴奋性的影响：心肌兴奋性大小主要与 Em－Et 间距长短有关。细胞外液钾浓度增高，静息期细胞内钾外流减少。在血钾浓度迅速轻度升高时，心肌细胞静息电位也轻度减小，引起兴奋所需的阈刺激也较小，即心肌兴奋性增高。当血钾浓度迅速显著升高时，由于静息电位过小，心肌兴奋性也将降低甚至消失。（2）对心肌传导性的影响：高钾血症时，由于静息电位减小，故动作电位 0 期（除极化）的幅度变小，速度减慢，因而兴奋的扩布减慢，即传导性降低。（3）对心肌自律性的影响：高钾血症时心肌细胞膜的钾通透性增高，故在到达最大复极电位后，细胞内钾的外流比正常时加快而钠内流相对减慢，因而自动去极化减慢，自律性降低。（4）对心肌收缩性的影响：高钾血症抑制钙内流，使心肌收缩性降低。

3. 答：在缺氧早期，（1）缺氧导致 PaO_2 的降低，可以刺激外周化学感受器（包括颈动脉体和主动脉体化学感受器），反射性地引起呼吸中枢兴奋。（2）缺氧导致酸性产物增多，也可以刺激外周和中枢化学感受器，兴奋呼吸中枢；使呼吸加深加快，增加肺通气量，这是一种代偿性反应。在缺氧晚期，随着缺氧程度的加重和时间的延长，缺氧直接抑制呼吸中枢，造成呼吸抑制，使呼吸减弱、减慢，甚至于停止。

4. 答：模型复制方法：（1）称重、固定、麻醉（1％普鲁卡因局麻）。（2）腹部手术：结扎肝右中叶、左中叶、左外侧叶，造成肝解毒功能急剧降低。（3）十二指肠插管。（4）给药：经十二指肠插管注入复方氯化铵溶液，5 ml/kg 体重，导致肠道中氨生成增多并吸收入血，引起家兔血氨迅速升高。

动物表现：兴奋性先增高后降低、角膜反射先灵敏后迟钝、扑翼样震颤、抽搐、肌肉震颤、肌肉痉挛、二便失禁、角弓反张、昏迷。

5. 答：腹部 1％普鲁卡因局部麻醉。因为肝性脑病实验中要观察的是氨对中枢神经系统的作用，如果采用全麻，中枢会受到抑制，不易观察中枢神经系统的表现，所以必须保证在整个实验过程中动物处于清醒状态。

（李　颖　杨秀红）

习 题 五

一、填空题

1. 硫酸镁口服给药，在胃肠道内发挥其_____作用，皮下注射给药则出现_____、_____，直至全身麻醉作用。
2. 可产生明显首关消除的给药途径是_____。
3. 浓度为 20% 的硫酸镁表示的含义是_____。
4. 镇痛药物实验方法有_____、_____、_____、_____。
5. 热板法测定药物的镇痛作用实验中，热板仪温度设定为_____。
6. 阿司匹林的药理作用是_____、_____、_____和_____等药理作用。
7. 镇痛药包括_____和_____。
8. 阿司匹林镇痛作用部位主要在_____，通过抑制炎症介质_____的合成，起到镇痛作用。
9. 曲马多属于_____，镇痛部位在_____；赖氨匹林属于_____，镇痛部位在_____。
10. 热板法测定药物的镇痛作用实验中，一般选择正常痛阈值为_____、性别为_____性的小鼠进行实验，小鼠疼痛表现是_____。
11. 小鼠腹腔注射醋酸引起疼痛的实验方法为_____，疼痛指标为_____。

二、单项选择题

1. 小白鼠灌胃给药时，一次给药量约为
   A. 0.1～0.2 ml/10 g
   B. 0.4～0.5 ml/10 g
   C. 0.6～0.7 ml/10 g
   D. 0.8～0.9 ml/10 g
2. 与药物效应强弱有关的药动学过程是
   A. 药物吸收的速度
   B. 药物吸收的程度
   C. 药物消除的速度
   D. 血药浓度维持的时间
3. 硫酸镁可因给药途径不同而产生不同的药理作用，口服后的作用是
   A. 降压抗惊厥　　　　B. 降压镇痛
   C. 导泻利胆　　　　　D. 舒张血管
4. 与血药浓度的高低无关的因素是
   A. 用药剂量　　　　　B. 体内分布

   C. 肝代谢　　　　　　D. 体温
5. 下列哪种给药途径，药物首关消除最明显
   A. 口服给药　　　　　B. 舌下给药
   C. 皮下注射　　　　　D. 静脉注射
6. 下列给药途径中，根据药效产生快慢关系，一般情况下，由快到慢的顺序为
   A. 静脉注射-肌内注射-皮下注射-口服
   B. 静脉注射-皮下注射-肌内注射-口服
   C. 静脉注射-肌内注射-口服-皮下注射
   D. 口服-肌内注射-皮下注射-静脉注射
7. 在小鼠腹腔注射中，下列说法错误的是
   A. 注射时应从左下腹或右下腹进针，避开膀胱
   B. 进针时以 60°角直接刺入腹腔
   C. 在给药前应回抽，判断有无血液或尿液

D. 腹腔注射给药量一般为 0.1～0.2 ml/10 g

8. 药物效应的强弱取决于

A. 吸收速度　　　　　B. 消除速度

C. 血浆蛋白结合率　　D. 剂量的大小

三、多项选择题

1. 下列说法正确的是

A. 在一定剂量范围内，随着给药剂量的加大，药物效应逐渐增强

B. 随着给药剂量的加大，药物的性质可能发生改变

C. 随着给药剂量的加大，药物效应会无限制的增强

D. 随着给药剂量的加大，药物效应逐渐增强，但药物作用的性质不会改变

2. 动物编号常用的方法有

A. 挂牌法　　　　　B. 染色法

C. 烙印法　　　　　D. 耳孔法

3. 水合氯醛的药理作用有

A. 镇静　　　　　　B. 催眠

C. 抗惊厥　　　　　D. 麻醉

4. 实验动物注射给药途径有

A. 皮下注射　　　　B. 腹腔注射

C. 肌内注射　　　　D. 静脉注射

5. 小鼠皮下注射硫酸镁可以产生抗惊厥作用，其原因为

A. 硫酸镁能抑制中枢和外周神经系统，使骨骼肌和血管平滑肌松弛

B. 对神经元有膜稳定作用

C. Mg^{2+} 可拮抗 Ca^{2+} 的作用，干扰 Ca^{2+} 的释放

D. 可以阻断多巴胺受体

6. 可能产生首关消除的给药途径有

A. 灌胃　　　　　　B. 腹腔注射

C. 静脉注射　　　　D. 皮下注射

7. 机能实验中，有关药物的配制方法以及常用动物给药量的表示方法正确的是

A. 药品常配成百分浓度（%）

B. 百分浓度的含义是每 100 ml 溶液中含多少克药物

C. 动物常按体重给药

D. 大鼠常按每 10 g 体重给药

8. 小鼠扭体反应表现为

A. 腰腹部内凹　　　　B. 弓腰

C. 躯体与后腿伸张　　D. 躯体与后肢卷曲

9. 在使用扭体法进行的镇痛实验中，下列说法正确的是

A. 为减少个体差异对实验结果造成的影响，应汇总全班实验结果进行统计

B. 扭体反应次数越多说明小鼠疼痛越明显

C. 使用赖氨匹林后所有小鼠均不再出现扭体反应

D. 冰醋酸通过刺激腹膜引起小鼠剧烈疼痛

10. 热板法实验中，下列描述正确的是

A. 测定痛反应时一旦小鼠出现典型痛反应，应立即移开，避免烫伤小鼠

B. 不能选用雄性小鼠

C. 室温应保持在 15～20 ℃为宜

D. 只有舔后足才作为疼痛的指标

11. 扭体法实验中，下列描述正确的是

A. 醋酸溶液需临时配制，如放置过久，作用明显减弱

B. 化学刺激法应在室温 20 ℃左右进行，温度过低时小白鼠扭体次数减少

C. 小白鼠体重应在 22～26 g，体重过轻，扭体反应出现率亦低

D. 应汇总全班实验结果计算镇痛百分率

四、判断题

( ) 1. 随着给药剂量的加大，药物效应会无限制的增强。
( ) 2. 硫酸镁抗惊厥作用的机理为可以阻断多巴胺受体。
( ) 3. 大白鼠给药量一般按每 100 g 体重给多少克药物。
( ) 4. 小白鼠灌胃给药时，一次给药量最多不能超过 5 ml。
( ) 5. 小白鼠腹腔注射，针尖与皮肤所成角度应为 60°。
( ) 6. 热板法实验测定痛反应时，一旦出现典型的疼痛症状，即应立即移开热板仪以免烫伤。
( ) 7. 小白鼠体重应在 15～18 g，体重过重，扭体反应出现率低。
( ) 8. 化学刺激法应在室温 20 ℃左右进行，温度过低时小白鼠扭体次数减少。
( ) 9. 曲马多和赖氨匹林可提高痛阈，推迟小鼠疼痛反应出现的时间。
( ) 10. 痛阈值是从小鼠放在热板仪上到出现舔后足的时间。
( ) 11. 一般选择痛阈值在 30～60 s 小鼠进行实验。
( ) 12. 热板法实验一般选择雄性小鼠，因雌性小鼠对热刺激敏感而影响实验结果。
( ) 13. 镇痛药物实验中给予生理盐水的目的是观察其是否具有镇痛作用。

五、简答题

1. 小鼠经灌胃或皮下注射给予 10％硫酸镁溶液后，各有何表现？机制是什么？
2. 腹腔注射 1％、10％水合氯醛，小鼠反应有何不同？机制是什么？
3. 热板法镇痛药物实验，曲马多和赖氨匹林哪个镇痛效果更好？为什么？
4. 中枢性镇痛药及外周镇痛药的镇痛机制分别是什么？

习题五参考答案

一、填空题

1. 导泻利胆　降压　抗惊厥（肌松）
2. 口服给药
3. 100 ml 溶液中含有 20 g 硫酸镁
4. 机械刺激法　电刺激法　热刺激法　化学刺激法
5. （55±0.5）℃
6. 解热　镇痛　抗炎抗风湿　抑制血小板聚集
7. 中枢性镇痛药　外周性镇痛药
8. 外周　前列腺素
9. 中枢性镇痛药　中枢　外周性镇痛药　外周
10. 5～30 s　雌　舔后足

11. 扭体法　扭体反应

二、单项选择题

1. A　2. B　3. C　4. D　5. A　6. A　7. B　8. D

三、多项选择题

1. AB　2. ABCD　3. ABCD　4. ABCD　5. AC　6. AB　7. ABC　8. ABC
9. ABD　10. ABCD　11. ABCD

四、判断题

1. ×　2. ×　3. √　4. ×　5. ×　6. √　7. ×　8. √　9. √　10. √　11. ×
12. ×　13. ×

五、简答题

1. 答：（1）灌胃硫酸镁，翻正反射存在有时可见大便增多。因口服硫酸镁不易被吸收，在肠腔内形成一种高渗透压，而阻碍水分的吸收，导致泻下作用。（2）注射 10％ 硫酸镁，小鼠嗜睡、翻正反射消失。硫酸镁能抑制中枢和外周神经系统，使骨骼肌松弛。机理：Mg^{2+} 和 Ca^{2+} 化学性质相似，可以特异性的竞争 Ca^{2+} 的受点，拮抗 Ca^{2+} 的作用，使 Ca^{2+} 参与的神经肌接头处 ACh 的释放减少，骨骼肌松弛；且可作用于中枢神经系统，抑制中枢，引起感觉和意识消失，故小鼠翻正反射消失。

2. 答：腹腔注射 1％ 水合氯醛，小鼠表现活动减少，翻正反射存在；10％ 水合氯醛表现为嗜睡，翻正反射消失，甚至死亡。水合氯醛为镇静催眠药，小剂量时表现为镇静，引起安静和嗜睡，随着剂量加大表现为催眠、抗惊厥和麻醉作用。

3. 答：曲马多的镇痛效果好于赖氨匹林。因为曲马多为中枢性镇痛药，通过与阿片受体结合并激动阿片受体，从而阻断痛觉冲动的传导过程，产生强大的镇痛作用；赖氨匹林为解热镇痛药，镇痛部位在外周，通过抑制前列腺素合成酶，使前列腺素的合成减少而产生镇痛作用。

4. 答：中枢性镇痛药：主要作用于中枢神经系统，选择性地消除或缓解痛觉的药物，可激动阿片受体，模拟内源性阿片肽，阻断痛觉传导通路产生镇痛作用。

外周镇痛药：镇痛作用在外周，它主要通过抑制前列腺素合成酶，使致痛物质前列腺素合成减少而减轻疼痛。

（张　娜　杨秀红）

习 题 六

一、填空题

1. 被动转运即药物从浓度_____的一侧向_____的一侧扩散，不消耗_____，不需_____参与，不受_____和_____的影响。

2. 水杨酸钠为_____性（酸碱性）药物。当尿液呈酸性时，水杨酸钠解离型_____，脂溶性_____，所以，药物通过细胞膜也越_____。

3. "尿液 pH 对药物排泄的影响"实验可得到的结论是_____。

4. 离子障原理为_____。

5. 激动药为既有_____又有_____的药物，它们能与受体结合并激动受体而产生效应。

6. 根据拮抗药与受体结合是否具有可逆性而将其分为_____和_____两类。

7. 肠道平滑肌上存在_____、_____、_____、_____及 5-羟色胺受体等多种受体。

8. M 胆碱受体和 H_1 受体兴奋时，肠平滑肌_____；α 受体和 β 受体兴奋时，肠平滑肌_____。

9. 放入恒温平滑肌槽内肠管标本应_____悬挂。

10. 竞争性拮抗药的作用强度常用_____表示，其值_____，拮抗作用越强。

二、单项选择题

1. 大多数药物跨膜转运的方式是
   A. 滤过　　　　　B. 胞饮
   C. 易化扩散　　　D. 简单扩散

2. 在酸性尿液中，弱酸性药物
   A. 解离多，重吸收的多，排泄慢
   B. 解离少，重吸收的多，排泄慢
   C. 解离少，重吸收的少，排泄快
   D. 解离少，重吸收的多，排泄快

3. 在碱性尿液中，弱酸性药物
   A. 解离少，重吸收的多，排泄慢
   B. 解离多，重吸收的少，排泄快
   C. 解离少，重吸收的多，排泄快
   D. 解离多，重吸收的多，排泄慢

4. 弱碱性药物与抗酸药同服，比单独服用该药
   A. 在胃中解离增多，自胃吸收增多
   B. 在胃中解离减少，自胃吸收增多
   C. 在胃中解离减少，自胃吸收减少
   D. 在胃中解离增多，自胃吸收减少

5. 受体阻断药（拮抗药）的特点是
   A. 有亲和力，无内在活性
   B. 有亲和力，有内在活性
   C. 有亲和力，有较弱内在活性
   D. 无亲和力，有内在活性

6. H_1 受体阻断剂对哪种病最有效
   A. 支气管哮喘　　B. 皮肤黏膜过敏症状
   C. 过敏性休克　　D. 过敏性紫癜

7. 离体豚鼠肠管应放在
   A. 乐氏液　　　　B. 台氏液
   C. 林格液　　　　D. 改良的克氏液

8. 加入氯化钡，豚鼠肠平滑肌发生何变化
   A. 肠平滑肌松弛
   B. 肠平滑肌先收缩，后松弛
   C. 肠平滑肌收缩

D. 肠平滑肌先松弛，后收缩

放入_____冲洗

9. 取豚鼠肠管部位最好选择

    A. 十二指肠   B. 大肠

    C. 远端回肠   D. 空肠

10. 从豚鼠腹腔取出的 5～6 cm 肠管应首先

A. 凉的营养液再剪成小段

B. 温的营养液再剪成小段

C. 凉的生理盐水再剪成小段

D. 温的生理盐水再剪成小段

三、多项选择题

1. 药物主动转运的特点是

    A. 需要消耗能量

    B. 可受其他药物的干扰

    C. 有化学结构特异性

    D. 转运速度有饱和限制

2. 药物的排泄过程

    A. 极性大的药物在肾小管重吸收少

    B. 酸性药物在碱性尿液中解离少，排泄慢

    C. 脂溶性高的药物在肾小管重吸收多

    D. 解离度大的药物重吸收少，易于排泄

3. 影响大多数药物从肾排泄速度的因素有

    A. 药物极性   B. 尿液 pH

    C. 肾功能状况   D. 给药剂量

4. 豚鼠肠管离体组织体外存活条件是

    A. $T = (38 \pm 0.5)℃$ B. 改良克氏液

    C. 自然给氧   D. 改良林格液

5. 对苯海拉明的描述，哪项是正确的

    A. 可用于晕动病引起的呕吐

B. 可用于治疗荨麻疹

C. 是 H_1 受体阻断剂

D. 可治疗胃和十二指肠溃疡

6. 竞争性拮抗药具有如下特点

    A. 能与激动药竞争相同受体

    B. 激动药增加剂量时，仍能达到原效应

    C. 能抑制激动药的最大效能

    D. 使激动药量效曲线平行右移

7. H_1 受体阻断剂的各项叙述，正确的是

    A. 主要用于治疗变态反应性疾病

    B. 主要代表药有法莫替丁

    C. 可用于治疗晕动病引起的呕吐

    D. 最常见的不良反应是中枢抑制现象

8. 非竞争性拮抗药的特点包括

    A. 与受体结合非常牢固

    B. 与受体结合是不可逆的

    C. 与受体结合后分离很慢

    D. 降低激动剂最大效能

四、判断题

（　）1. 水杨酸钠在碱性尿液中排泄增加。

（　）2. 当弱酸性药物中毒时，可用 NaOH 碱化尿液。

（　）3. 当弱酸性药物中毒时，可用稀 HCl 酸化尿液。

（　）4. 水杨酸钠在碱性尿液中，主要以离子状态存在。

（　）5. 天然组胺以无活性形式存在，在组织损伤、炎症、神经刺激等条件下，以活性形式释放。

（　）6. "苯海拉明对组胺的竞争性拮抗作用"实验中，给药时可将药液直接滴加到肠管上，才能起到更好的实验效果。

（　）7. "苯海拉明对组胺的竞争性拮抗作用"实验中，每次加药前，均应冲洗肠管，待肠管恢复正常运动后再观察下一项目。

（　）8.“苯海拉明对组胺的竞争性拮抗作用”实验中，开始应先给予乌拉坦麻醉豚鼠，再取出肠管。

（　）9.组胺可用于检查胃酸分泌功能。

（　）10.苯海拉明能与组胺竞争 H_1 受体，使组胺不能同 H_1 受体结合而起拮抗作用。

五、简答题

1.改变尿液的 pH 对临床用药有何指导意义？

2.给予苯海拉明后再给予不同浓度组胺，离体肠平滑肌收缩曲线如何变化？机制是什么？

3.组胺、氯化钡分别作用于离体回肠后，肠平滑肌收缩曲线如何变化？作用机制有何不同？

习题六参考答案

一、填空题

1.高　低　能量　酶或载体　饱和　竞争

2.弱酸　减少　增强　多

3.水杨酸钠等弱酸性药物在碱性环境中重吸收少，排泄多；在酸性环境中重吸收多，排泄少

4.分子型药物易跨膜转运，离子型药物不易跨膜转运

5.亲和力　内在活性

6.竞争性拮抗药　非竞争性拮抗药

7.M受体　α受体　β受体　组胺受体

8.收缩　松弛

9.上下两端呈对角线

10.拮抗参数（pA_2）　越大

二、单项选择题

1.D　2.B　3.B　4.B　5.A　6.B　7.D　8.C　9.C　10.A

三、多项选择题

1.ABCD　2.ACD　3.ABCD　4.ABC　5.ABC　6.ABD　7.ACD　8.ABCD

四、判断题

1.√　2.×　3.×　4.√　5.√　6.×　7.√　8.×　9.√　10.√

五、简答题

1. 答：临床上，可以通过改变尿液的 pH 加速药物的排泄，解救药物中毒。当弱酸性药物中毒时，可用 $NaHCO_3$ 碱化尿液。因为当用 $NaHCO_3$ 碱化尿液时，会使弱酸性药物的解离型增多，所以重吸收减少，排泄增加。相反，当弱碱性药物中毒时，可用 NH_4Cl 酸化尿液。因为当用 NH_4Cl 酸化尿液时，会使弱碱性药物的解离型增多，所以，重吸收减少，排泄增加。

2. 答：给予苯海拉明后给予低浓度组胺，肠平滑肌收缩可能不出现增强表现，因为苯海拉明为 H_1 受体阻断药，组胺收缩肠平滑肌的作用可能完全被阻断；但随着组胺剂量增大，与苯海拉明争夺更多受体，引起肠平滑肌收缩加强。

3. 答：组胺可激动肠 H_1 受体，引起肠平滑肌收缩加强。原因：通过 IP_3、DAG 等信使分子介导，产生支气管与胃肠道平滑肌兴奋，引起肠平滑肌收缩加强。氯化钡使肠平滑肌收缩增强，呈强直性收缩。原因：Ba^{2+} 和 Ca^{2+} 化学性质相似，直接作用于肠平滑肌，使肠平滑肌呈强直性收缩。

（朱丽艳　杨秀红）

习 题 七

一、填空题

1. 可同时激动 α、β 受体的药物是_____，主要激动 α 受体的药物是_____，主要激动 β 受体的药物是_____。

2. 去甲肾上腺素引起的血压变化是收缩压_____，舒张压_____。

3. 异丙肾上腺素激动 β_2 受体产生的血管效应是_____。

4. 酚妥拉明为_____受体阻断剂，引起的血压变化是_____。

5. 有机磷酸酯类主要经过_____、_____、_____三条途径吸收，主要由_____排出体外。

6. 有机磷中毒时给予阿托品的原则是_____、_____、_____、_____。

7. 有机磷中毒时常用的解救药物是_____、_____。

8. 有机磷酸酯类中毒可观察_____、_____、_____、_____、_____指标。

9. 血胆碱酯酶活力正常值为_____；有机磷酸酯类轻度中毒为_____；中度中毒为_____；重度中毒为_____。

10. 有机磷酸酯类急性中毒的治疗原则有两方面：_____和_____。

二、单项选择题

1. 去甲肾上腺素对体内哪些部位的缩血管作用最强
   A. 肾血管　　　　　B. 肝、肠系膜血管
   C. 骨骼肌血管　　　D. 皮肤、黏膜血管

2. 肾上腺素作用最明显的部位是
   A. 胃肠道和膀胱　　B. 心血管
   C. 支气管　　　　　D. 眼睛

3. 异丙肾上腺素激动 β 受体产生的血管效应是
   A. 肾血管收缩　　　B. 脑血管收缩
   C. 骨骼肌血管扩张　D. 冠脉收缩

4. 异丙肾上腺素的主要药理作用有
   A. 兴奋心脏，升高收缩压和舒张压
   B. 抑制心脏，升高收缩压和降低舒张压
   C. 兴奋心脏，降低收缩压和升高舒张压
   D. 兴奋心脏，升高收缩压和降低舒张压

5. 给家兔静脉注射某药可引起血压升高，如预先给予酚妥拉明后，再注射该药时，则引起血压明显下降；但是如果预先注射普萘洛尔后再注射该药则引起血压上升，此药可能是
   A. 麻黄碱　　　　　B. 异丙肾上腺素
   C. 肾上腺素　　　　D. 去甲肾上腺素

6. 有机磷酸酯类中毒的原理是

   A. 胆碱酯酶失活
   B. 磷酰化胆碱酯酶减少
   C. 胆碱酯酶活性增强
   D. 交感神经兴奋

7. 急性有机磷中毒最主要的死因是
   A. 中毒性休克　　　B. 急性肾功能衰竭
   C. 呼吸衰竭　　　　D. 脑水肿

8. 重度有机磷中毒的表现，下列组合哪项是正确的
   A. 瞳孔明显缩小、视力模糊、大汗、肌无力
   B. 瞳孔明显扩大、视力模糊、大汗、肌无力
   C. 瞳孔明显扩大、视力模糊、大汗、肌张力增强
   D. 瞳孔明显缩小、视力模糊、大汗、肌张力不变

9. 有机磷中毒 N 样症状是
   A. 肌肉震颤　　　　B. 瞳孔减小
   C. 恶心呕吐　　　　D. 大汗淋漓

10. 碘解磷定对下列哪种药物中毒无效
    A. 内吸磷　　　　　B. 马拉硫磷
    C. 敌百虫　　　　　D. 乐果

三、多项选择题

1. 家兔耳缘静脉注射大剂量的肾上腺素后，引起的血压变化是
   A. 给药初期，舒张压、收缩压均升高
   B. 给药初期，舒张压降低、收缩压升高
   C. 给药后期，舒张压、收缩压均降低
   D. 给药后期，舒张压降低、收缩压升高

2. 下列存在于体内的拟交感胺类物质有
   A. 多巴胺　　　　　B. 异丙肾上腺素
   C. 肾上腺素　　　　D. 去甲肾上腺素

3. 去甲肾上腺素与肾上腺素相比，前者的特

点是
   A. 收缩血管及升压作用强
   B. 扩张支气管作用弱
   C. 对机体代谢影响小
   D. 对心脏兴奋作用弱

4. 异丙肾上腺素、肾上腺素、去甲肾上腺素共同具有的作用是
   A. 扩张骨骼肌血管
   B. 降低外周阻力
   C. 增加心肌收缩力

D. 升高收缩压

5. 肾上腺素的 α、β 受体被激动时，产生的效应是
   A. 激动 α 受体，血管平滑肌收缩
   B. 激动 β_1 受体使心脏兴奋
   C. 激动 β_2 受体使支气管平滑肌、冠脉、骨骼肌血管收缩
   D. 激动 β_2 受体使支气管平滑肌舒张，冠脉、骨骼肌血管收缩

6. 碘解磷定治疗有机磷酸酯中毒的主要机制是
   A. 与结合在胆碱酯酶上的磷酰基结合生成磷酰化碘解磷定
   B. 与 M 受体结合，使其不受有机磷酸酯类抑制

C. 与胆碱酯酶结合，保护其不与有机磷酸酯类结合
D. 与游离的有机磷酸酯类结合，促进其排泄

7. 阿托品具有的作用是
   A. 瞳孔缩小
   B. 瞳孔散大
   C. 调节麻痹，视近物不清
   D. 降低眼内压

8. 对一口服有机磷农药中毒的患者，下列抢救措施中正确的是
   A. 迅速洗胃
   B. 吸氧
   C. 待阿托品疗效不好时，加用碘解磷定
   D. 及早、足量、反复注射阿托品

四、判断题

（　）1. 大剂量的肾上腺素引起血压先升高后降低。
（　）2. 去甲肾上腺素引起血压的变化是舒张压升高、收缩压降低。
（　）3. 去甲肾上腺素主要激动 α 受体，同时对 β_1 受体也可微弱的激动。
（　）4. 异丙肾上腺素引起血压的变化是舒张压、收缩压均升高。
（　）5. 碘解磷定是乐果中毒首选的解毒剂。
（　）6. 碘解磷定和阿托品为治疗机磷酸酯类中毒的特异性、高效能解毒药物。
（　）7. 有机磷酸酯类重度中毒主要表现为 M 样症状和 N 样症状。
（　）8. 阿托品救治有机磷酸酯类中毒应大量用药至阿托品化。
（　）9. 有机磷酸酯类中毒，必须马上用胆碱酯酶复活剂抢救，因为被抑制的胆碱酯酶很快老化。
（　）10. 由耳缘静脉推注碘解磷定时速度宜慢，不宜过快，以免药物本身的毒性引起家兔死亡。

五、简答题

1. 什么叫后 β 效应？
2. 给予酚妥拉明后再给予肾上腺素，家兔血压有何变化？机制是什么？
3. 有机磷酸酯类轻、中、重度中毒时临床症状是什么？
4. 为什么在使用 M 受体阻断剂时，又给予碘解磷定治疗有机磷酸酯类中毒？
5. 遇到敌百虫口服中毒的患者，应如何处理？

习题七参考答案

一、填空题

1. 肾上腺素　去甲肾上腺素　异丙肾上腺素
2. 升高　明显升高
3. 血管舒张
4. α　下降
5. 消化道　呼吸道　皮肤黏膜　肾
6. 联合用药　尽早用药　足量用药　重复用药
7. 阿托品　碘解磷定
8. 瞳孔大小　唾液分泌　肌张力　肌震颤　大小便　酶活性
9. 100%　70%～50%　50%～30%　30%以下
10. 迅速消除毒物　积极使用解毒药

二、单项选择题

1. D　2. B　3. C　4. D　5. C　6. A　7. C　8. A　9. A　10. D

三、多项选择题

1. AC　2. ACD　3. ABCD　4. CD　5. AB　6. AD　7. BC　8. ABD

四、判断题

1. √　2. ×　3. √　4. ×　5. ×　6. √　7. ×　8. √　9. √　10. √

五、简答题

1. 答：血压降低的效应也叫后 β 效应。大剂量的肾上腺素给药时，对血压的影响呈双相反应：血压先升高后降低。随着用药时间的延长，肾上腺素不断被代谢、排泄，肾上腺素的血药浓度逐渐降低，此时血压的表现是舒张压、收缩压均降低。原因是由于 β_2 受体对小剂量的肾上腺素敏感，所以主要表现为 β_2 受体被激动引起的血管舒张，舒张压降低；收缩压也降低的原因是由于血管舒张会引起回心血量减少，导致心输出量降低，所以收缩压下降。

2. 答：给予酚妥拉明后给予肾上腺素，血压可能不再升高而降低，出现肾上腺素翻转效应，酚妥拉明为 α 受体阻断药，而参与血管舒张有关的 β_2 受体未被阻断，故肾上腺素的血管收缩作用被取消，而血管舒张作用充分表现出来。

3. 答：轻度中毒：主要表现为 M 样症状，如瞳孔缩小、腺体分泌增多、呼吸困难、恶心呕吐、大小便失禁等。中度中毒：除 M 样症状外还有 N 样症状，表现为肌肉震颤、抽搐、肌张力降低等。重度中毒：除 M 样症状、N 样症状还有中枢神经系统症状，如头痛头晕、昏迷、呼吸肌麻痹、窒息等。

4. 答：单用 M 受体阻断剂（阿托品）能迅速缓解 M 样症状，但对抗 N_2 受体的兴奋作用差，不能有效抑制骨骼肌震颤，对中毒晚期的呼吸肌麻痹也无效，且无复活胆碱酯酶的作用，疗效不宜巩固。而胆碱酯酶复活药（碘解磷定）则对抑制骨骼肌震颤症状疗效较好，但对 M 样症状作用较弱。（由于碘解磷定不能直接对抗体内积聚的 ACh 的作用）。因此两药合用时有机磷酸酯类的中毒症状得到全面改善，疗效大大提高。故而临床对有机磷酸酯类中毒的抢救治疗以阿托品加胆碱酯酶复活药联合应用。

5. 答：（1）立即将患者移出现场，去除污染的衣物。（2）对皮肤吸收者，应用温水清洗皮肤。经口中毒者，应首先抽出胃液和毒物，并用微温的 1‰盐水反复洗胃，直至洗出液中不含农药味。（3）给予硫酸镁导泻。（4）采用阿托品与胆碱酯酶复活药并用。

（朱丽艳　杨秀红）

附　录

附表 1　用基础溶液配制生理溶液的配方
Tab. 1　Preparation of physiological solution with basic solution formula

成分	基础溶液浓度（g/100ml）	林格液（ml）	乐氏液（ml）	台氏液（ml）
氯化钠（NaCl）	20.0	32.5	45.0	40.0
氯化钾（KCl）	10.0	1.4	4.2	2.0
氯化钙（$CaCl_2$）	10.0	1.2	2.4	2.0
磷酸二氢钠（NaH_2PO_4）	1.0	1.0	—	5.0
氯化镁（$MgCl_2$）	5.0	—	—	2.0
碳酸氢钠（$NaHCO_3$）	5.0	4.0	2.0	20.0
加蒸馏水至		1000.0	1000.0	1000.0

附表 2　几种生理代用液中的固体成分的含量（单位：克）
Tab. 2　Content of solid in several physiological substitutes（unit：g）

成分	生理盐水		林格液		乐氏液	台氏液	克氏液
	两栖类	哺乳类	两栖类	哺乳类	哺乳类	哺乳类小肠	哺乳类
氯化钠（NaCl）	6.50	9.00	6.50	9.00	8.00	6.90
氯化钾（KCl）	—	—	0.14	0.42	0.20	0.35
氯化钙（$CaCl_2$）	—	—	0.12	0.24	0.20	0.28
碳酸氢钠（$NaHCO_3$）	—	—	0.20	0.10~0.30	1.00	2.10
磷酸二氢钠（NaH_2PO_4）	—	—	0.01	—	0.05	—
磷酸二氢钾（KH_2PO_4）	—	—	—	—	—	0.16
氯化镁（$MgCl_2$）	—	—	—	—	0.10	—
硫酸镁（$MgSO_4 \cdot 7H_2O$）	—	—	—	—	—	0.29
葡萄糖	—	—	2.00	1.00~1.50	1.00	2.00
加蒸馏水至	1000.00	1000.00	1000.00	1000.00	1000.00	1000.00

附表 3　常用实验动物的正常生理、生化指标

Tab. 3　Animal's normal physiological and biochemical index

	单位	狗	兔	豚鼠	大鼠	小鼠	蛙
体重(成年)	kg	6.0~15.0	1.5~3.0	0.5~0.9	180~250 (g)	20~25 (g)	30 (g)
体温	℃	37.3~38.8	37.7~38.8	37.3~39.5	38.5~39.5	37.0~39.0	变温动物
心率	次/分	90~130	150~240	144~300	286~500	520~780	30~60
呼吸	次/分	12~28	50~100	80~130	110~150	140~210	70~120（室温）
血压	kPa	16.0~21.3	10.7~17.3	9.3~10.7	13.3~17.3	13.3~13.6	2.66~8.0
总血量	占体重%	5.0~8.0	5.4	5.8	7.0	7.0	4.2~4.9
血红蛋白	g/L	130~200	124	130	160	112~160	72~105
红细胞	$\times10^{12}$/L	4~8	4~6.4	5	5.31~11	8~11	0.38~0.64
白细胞	$\times10^{9}$/L	5~15	3.8~12	8.0~10.0	5~25.6	7~15	2.41~39.1
血小板	$\times10^{9}$/L	200~900	126~300	54~100	430~1000	100~400	8.5~39
血糖（全血）	mmol/L	4.3~6.1	6.2~8.7	5.3~8.4	5.1~6.9	8.7~9.5	0.6~4.1
总蛋白	g/L	63~81	60~83	50~56	69~79	52~57	34.6~79
白蛋白	g/L	34~45	41~50	28~39	26~35	16~17	—
血清氯	mmol/L	104~117	92~112	94~110	94~110	109~118	—
血清钾	mmol/L	3.7~5.0	2.7~5.1	6.5~8.7	3.8~5.4	7.5~7.7	—
血清钠	mmol/L	129~149	155~165	158	126~155	145~161	—
尿量	L/24h	1~2	0.18~0.44	0.05	0.015	0.002	约1/3体重
尿比重	—	1.025	1.010~1.015	1.033~1.036	—	—	1.0015
尿酸	mg/100ml	1.7	2.6	2.5	2.5	6.0	
NPN	mg/100ml	1.7	2.6	2.5	2.5	6.0	—
寿命	年	10	7~8	6~8	2~3	2~3	10
性成熟	月	12	5~8	4~5	2~3	2~3	—

主要参考书目

1. 朱大年. 生理学. 7 版. 北京：人民卫生出版社，2008.

2. 金惠铭，王建枝. 病理生理学. 7 版. 北京：人民卫生出版社，2008.

3. 杨宝峰. 药理学. 7 版. 北京：人民卫生出版社，2008.

4. 张连元，杨林. 机能实验教程. 北京：人民军医出版社，2007.

5. 杨芳炬. 机能实验学. 北京：高等教育出版社，2010.

6. 白波，刘善庭. 医学机能学实验教程. 2 版. 北京：人民卫生出版社，2009.

7. 谢可鸣，茅彩萍，王国卿，蒋星红. 机能实验学. 2 版. 苏州：苏州大学出版社，2007.

8. 崔庚寅，解景田. 生理学实验释疑解难. 北京：科学出版社，2007.

9. 郝刚，李效义. 医学机能学实验教程. 北京大学医学出版社，2007：15 - 27.